Doctor Lois

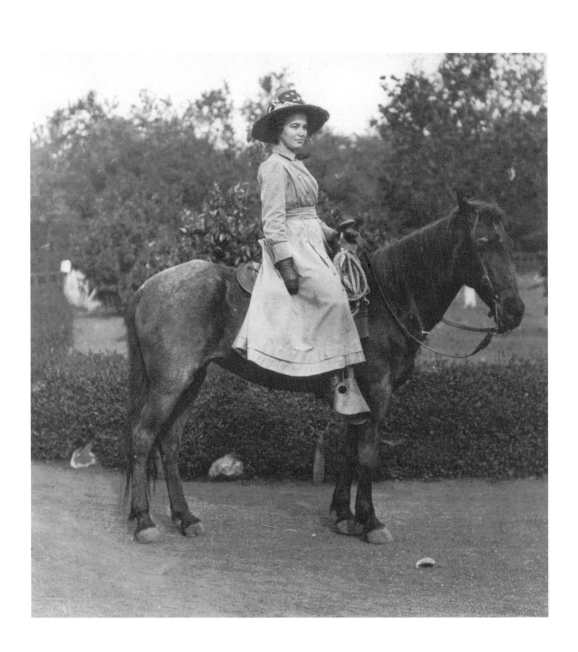

Doctor Lois

a Biography of

Lois Pendleton Todd, M.D.

1894–1968

by her daughter
Elinor Todd Christiansen, M.D.

Liibrary of Congress Catalog Card Number: 98-073984

ISBN: 1-889385-03-4 Paperback
ISBN: 1-889385-04-2 Hardcover

Cover and Book Design by:
Paulette Livers Lambert
4319 Snowberry Court
Boulder, Colorado 80304
(303) 444-9679

Book Editorial and Publishing by:

Alpenrose Press

Mary Ellen Gilliland
Alpenrose Press
P. O. Box 499
Silverthorne, Colorado 80498
(970) 468-6273

To Order This Book, Write:

Dr. Lois Book Offer
c/o Christiansen
4081 South Holly Street
Denver, Colorado 80111
(303) 756-4159

$24.95 in hardcover
$16.95 in quality paperback

PRINTED IN THE UNITED STATES OF AMERICA

Acknowledgments

I AM GRATEFUL to many sources for the information included in this biography and genealogy of my mother, Lois Pendleton Todd, M.D., including the stories she and her mother shared with me as I was growing up. My grandmother, Jessie Larimore Pendleton, was a diligent and meticulous parent who prepared family albums for each of her children. On Christmas 1917, Lois's parents presented her with a large photo album with over 200 pages of family pictures, all mounted, identified, and dated.

Lois kept her own photo albums during her college years and her years working in Tehchow. When my parents married, they took frequent photographs to send home to family members in America. In 1938, before leaving China, Lois compiled four to six small volumes of family pictures for each of her four children.

Alice Reed, who was Girls' School principal at Tehchow and house-mate of Lois from 1920 to 1927, typed weekly letters to her family at home in America. When I visited Alice at Pilgrim Place in Claremont, she was in her nineties and still keen, although frail. She kindly loaned to me her thick binder of letters to her family and answered many questions, sharing additional memories.

Uncle Morris Pendleton, Lois's younger brother, dictated many of his memories for me when he learned that I had embarked upon the project of writing the story of my mother's life. When Morris died, his long-time secretary and administrative assistant, Evelyn Andrade, sent to me the correspondence between Lois and Morris and also a box of family photographs that had been in storage.

Adaline Pendleton Satterthwaite, M.D., Lois's sister, kindly loaned me the binder of typed letters her mother wrote to friends in America during the two years they spent with Lois in Tehchow, China and Robert in Los Banos, the Philippines in 1926–1927.

My brothers shared with me copies of newspaper clippings and the Stanford University Faculty Senate Memorial Resolution on Dr. Lois Pendleton Todd. I appreciate the nudging of my siblings and nieces when I took a long break from this labor of love.

My friends' many words of encouragement have helped me to complete this project, which I began in 1985 after my first retirement. The first five years were devoted to research and compiling my mother's genealogy (see Family Foundations I and II.) Valuable sources included several books about early and late Pendletons and the *Sea Captains of Searsport*. A visit to the Penobscot Marine

Museum in Searsport in 1976 was extremely valuable. Lois's cousin Mary (Morris) Embleton, at the urging of Lois, wrote an 18 page genealogy of the Morris family after much research in the 1940's when she retired from teaching history and English.

I am grateful for the technical assistance my husband, Robert M. Christiansen, has provided from beginning to end.

My sincere gratitude goes to Mary Ellen Gilliland of Alpenrose Press, who worked with me as editor and publisher. She enabled my manuscript to become a book. My appreciation and gratitude also go to Paulette Livers Lambert, the very talented graphic designer who designed the the book's cover and interior. My sincere thanks go to my dear friend Velva (Peggy) Severson who kindly and patiently did the proof-reading for me. It has been a team effort.

Contents

Introduction

WHEN I RETIRED from my busy medical career I decided to write the biography of my mother, Lois Pendleton Todd, M.D. (1894–1968), who was such a wonderful role model for me. She successfully balanced a demanding medical career with raising four children. Few women in 1920 were as bright, well-educated, eager, well-trained in her chosen profession, highly motivated, dedicated, and courageous as Lois Pendleton, M.D., when she sailed for China to serve as physician and surgeon in a mission hospital in Shantung province, China.

My mother was a remarkable lady. She enjoyed a life full of adventure and challenge, joy and satisfaction. She studied and appreciated Chinese language and culture, threw all her energies into healing the sick and injured, enjoyed an avid sports life, raised four active children, traveled the globe, and never stopped touching individual lives. I want my children and their children to know the story of her life. Other family members and many outside the family will find the story of a young female surgeon who sailed for China in 1920 an interesting and inspiring story—a remarkable story of faith, courage, and achievement.

The story of her paternal and maternal ancestors illuminates who she was and the origins of her character traits: courage, love of adventure, eagerness to assume responsibility, desire to serve others, a sense of "calling," commitment, liberal and independent thinking, and an appreciation of nature, beauty, and music. You will find many examples of her character traits among the stories of her ancestors in Family Foundations I and II.

My hope is that the story of Doctor Lois will inspire future generations. She gave the gift of her life to me. I want to share that gift with you, my readers.

—*Elinor Todd Christiansen, M.D.*

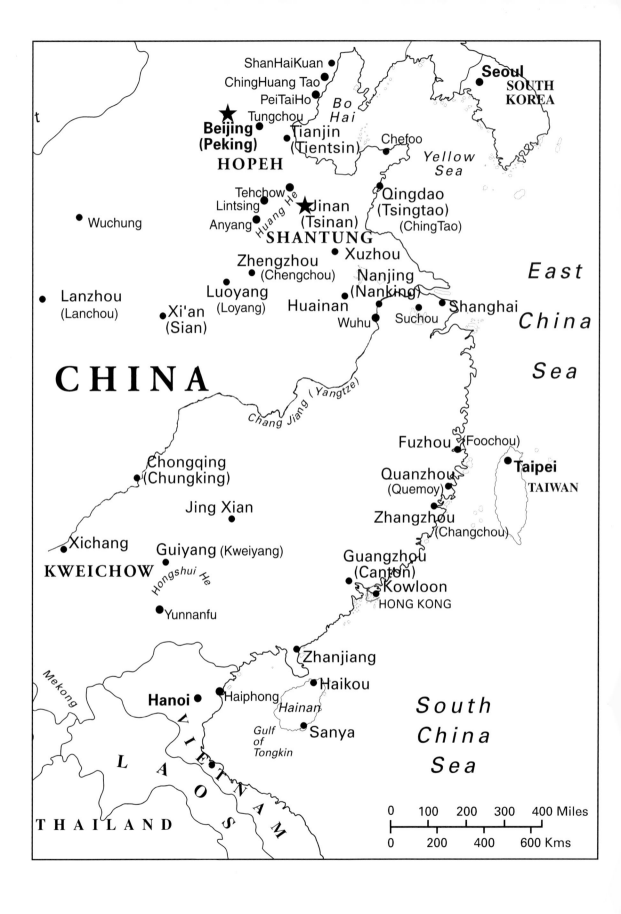

CHAPTER 1

Westward Move

John Louis Pendleton was born in Searsport, Maine, on July 24, 1866 the son of John Gilmore Pendleton, master mariner, and his second wife, Sarah E. Blanchard of Belfast, Maine. When steam-driven ships replaced sailing ships in the 1870's, sea captains became merchants of durable goods, hardware, and ship chandlery. As a result, John Louis Pendleton entered the hardware business, instead of being a sea captain sailing clipper ships around the world as generations of his family had done. His first job was in a hardware store in Belfast, Maine.

MINNESOTA

J. Louis Pendleton (French pronunciation "Louie") moved west at age 21 to work at the Morrison Hardware Company, a business owned by his elder sister Evelyn Morrison and her husband in Minneapolis, Minnesota. He lived at a boarding house, as was common for single persons in those days, which was operated by a widow named Adaline Ann Larimore, a former school teacher from Bryan, Ohio.

After the death of her husband, Dr. Andrew Jackson Larimore, a beloved physician in Bryan, Adaline Larimore moved northwest to Minneapolis with her three children from this marriage: John, Jessie, and Jennie. John studied law at University of Minnesota and Jessie became a school teacher at age 18.

Louis soon fell in love with Adaline Larimore's daughter, Jessie. The young hardware salesman from Maine and Jessie Larimore were both active in

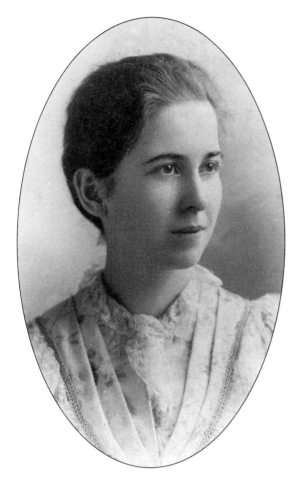

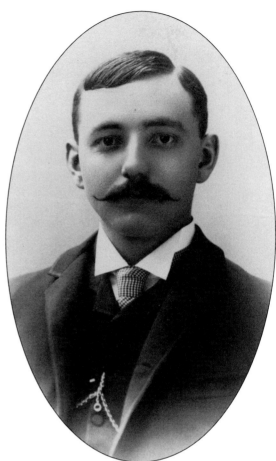

Jessie Larimore Pendleton
age 22, mother of Lois.

John Louis Pendleton
age 26, father of Lois.

the Christian Endeavor Youth Group of Plymouth Congregational Church and married in this church on June 25, 1889. Their first child, Robert Larimore Pendleton, was born June 25, 1890 on his parents' first wedding anniversary. Their second child, Lois Pendleton, was born April 14, 1894 in their home at 2100 Bryant Avenue on the south side of Minneapolis.

J. Louis Pendleton's work as a hardware salesman proved very strenuous with long hours. In those days on the frontier, Minneapolis hardware stores were open from 7:00 AM to 6:00 PM six days a week and "on call" on Sunday. Louis worked with such purpose, zeal, and effort, that his health eventually broke and he was forced to give up his job with Morrison Hardware. His physician advised him to move west to California for a milder climate.

CALIFORNIA

In 1895 Louis and Jessie moved west by train to Saratoga, California, with their son Robert age five and infant daughter Lois age one, to establish their home. Saratoga was a new town with 250 families and a Congregational Church, located along the western edge of Santa Clara valley, a region being developed for fruit orchards: prunes, apricots, peaches, pears, cherries, and grapes.

It was a leap of faith, moving to the unknown frontier. When God counseled Abraham to leave his own country and go in pilgrimage into the land which God had shown him, the "Land of Promise", he went with faith and trust in God. Similarly, Louis and Jessie moved west on the advice of his physician, into the great unknown, with faith and trust that God would be with them.

Santa Clara valley looked like a "garden of Eden" to this young family from Minneapolis. They settled in Saratoga, purchased ten acres of land south of town, planted a prune orchard, built their home, and raised their family here for the next eighteen years.

To supplement the orchard income, J. Louis became a traveling hardware salesman, building upon his earlier experience. He made three trips per year, each lasting two months, to all major cities west of the Mississippi River, including Omaha, Kansas City, El Paso, Denver, Salt Lake City, and Spokane. Prior to his departure from Minneapolis for sunny California, he had lined up a number of wholesale products to sell to hardware stores so that he, with a large territory west of Minneapolis, could make a living as a "drummer" (drumming up business), now known as a "sales engineer".

House in Minneapolis where Lois was born April 14, 1894.

During the six months at home he managed the prune ranch and served as county road commissioner. Both Louis and Jessie were actively involved in civic organizations and most particularly in the Saratoga Congregational Church. The family thrived and prospered in Saratoga.

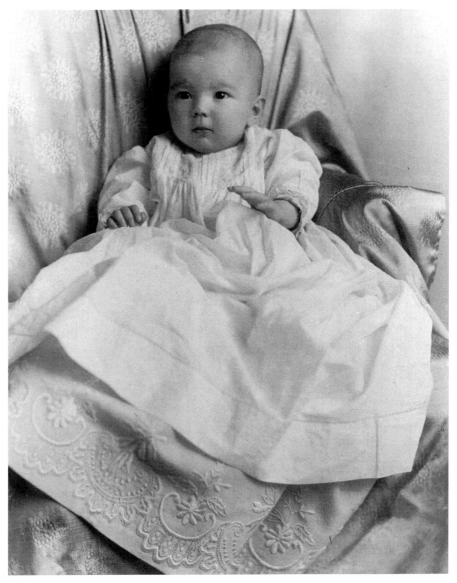

Lois age 5 months, Sept. 1894.

CHAPTER 2

Saratoga Childhood

Soon after arriving in Saratoga, John Louis Pendleton returned home one day after an outing to see the village; with excitement and pleasure he told his wife, Jessie, that he had just purchased a cemetery plot! Jessie was dismayed. How could he decide to buy a cemetery plot before they had a home or could

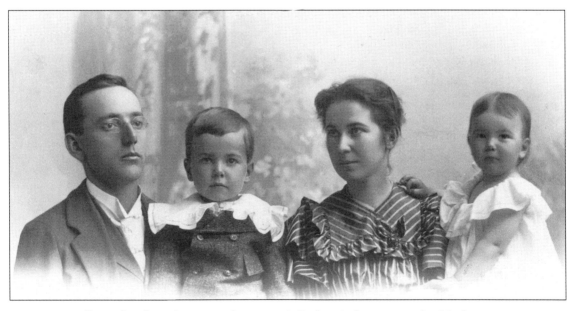

Pendleton family in Saratoga, Sept. 1895: Father, Robert age 5 1/2, Mother and Lois age 1 1/2.

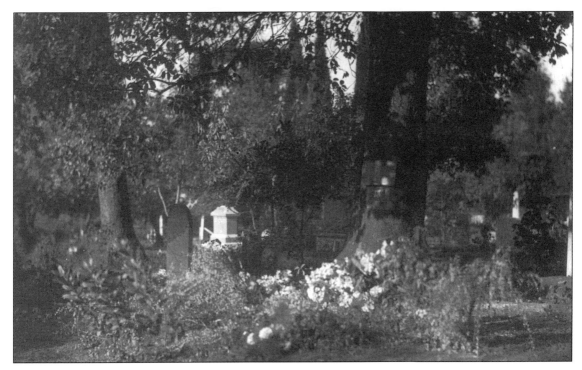

Madronia tree on Pendleton plot in Saratoga's Madronia Cemetery.
Below: Neighborhood children in Saratoga, June 1897: Mills Waterhouse,
Robert age 7, Arthur Foster, Clark Waterhouse age 4 and Lois age 3.

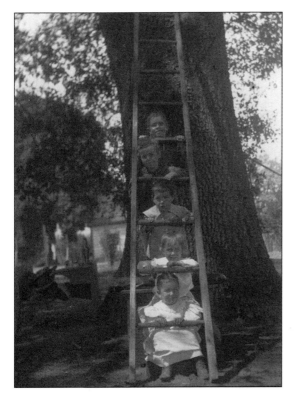

even afford to buy a milk cow to feed their little ones? Jessie cried with disappointment, but Louis went on to explain how he came across land being cleared for the beautiful new Madronia Cemetery on the west side of town at Sixth and Oak Streets.

Louis had an unusual fondness for trees and this area had stolen his heart with its many beautiful madronia trees (Arbutus Menziesii), smooth red trunks crowned by glossy dark green leaves. While admiring the beautiful madronias he met Frank Farwell, secretary and treasurer of the Madronia Cemetery Association, and Louis immediately arranged to purchase the plot on which the largest and most beautiful madronia tree stood.

(Later he bought the adjacent plot for family burials.) He fully expected Jessie to share his enthusiasm over acquiring this treasure for the family.

Frank Farwell soon showed John Louis Pendleton homesites and ten acre plots of land for sale for prune orchards about a mile south of Saratoga village, along the Saratoga to Los Gatos road. Louis selected ten acres on Farwell Avenue at the bend in the road, right across the road from Frank and Jennie Farwell's beautiful estate, Bella Vista.

Easy terms were arranged and Louis built a two story home for his family, along with a water tower, barn, and fruit house on

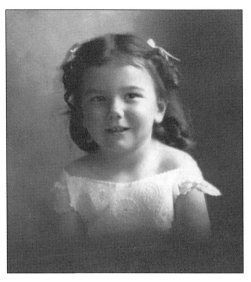

Lois age 3 1/2, Oct. 1897.
Below: Robert age 9 and Lois age 5
riding their donkey, "Topsy" in 1899.

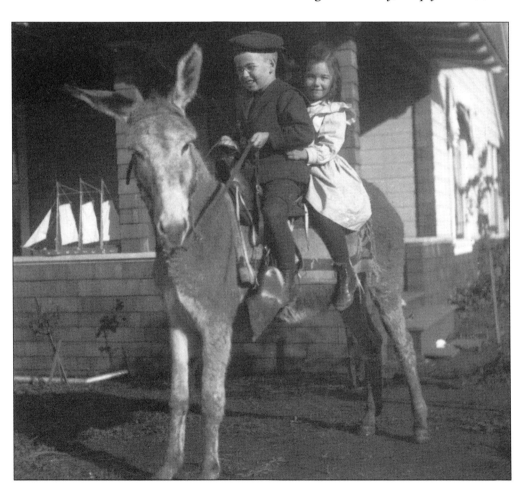

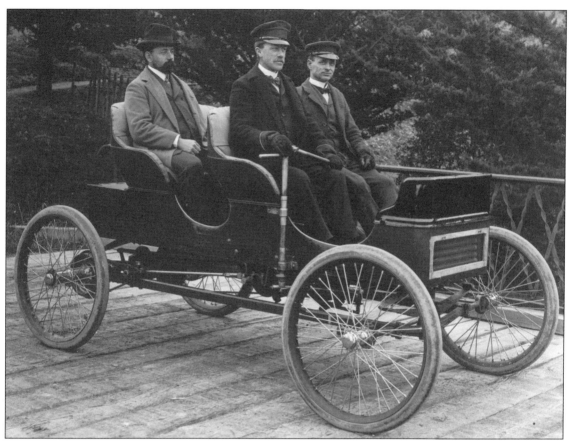

Father J. L. Pendleton (on left) riding in electric automobile made in San Jose, 1901.
Below: Lois and her friends Mills and Clark Waterhouse playing "Spanish War" in Farwell
Glen, 1902.

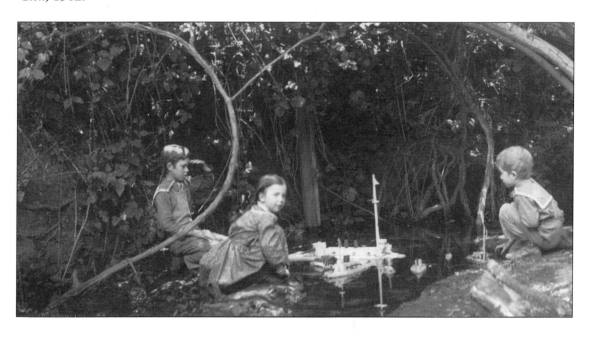

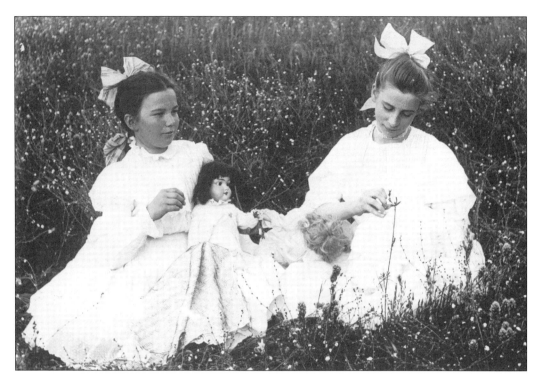

Lois and her friend Lottie Lake playing with dolls in meadow of forget-me-nots in Farwell Glen.
Below: Lois and her friend Lottie fishing in Wild-Cat Creek in Farwell Glen.

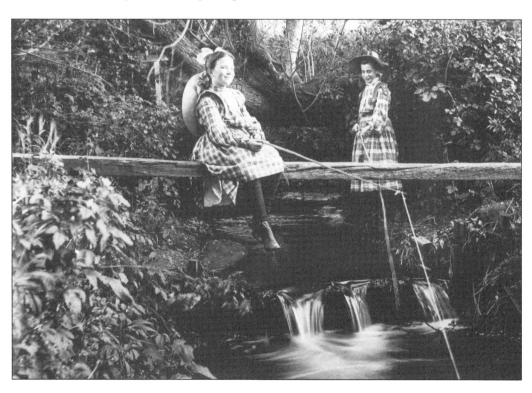

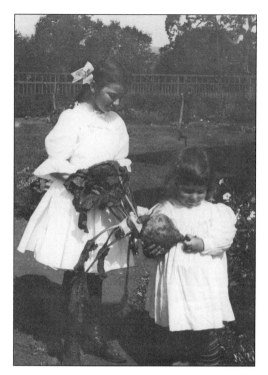

one acre. He cleared the remaining nine acres for planting a prune orchard; this remained under the control of the company (Saratoga Village Improvement Association) until the orchard became fruit bearing and final payments were made. With the generous help of new friends and neighbors the Pendleton family was soon established in Saratoga. They became active members of the Congregational Church and friendships grew.

Lois age 9 and brother Morris age 2 with giant beet from their garden in Saratoga. Below: Pendleton family home on Farwell Avenue with water tank behind house and bedroom for Lois under the water tank.

PENDLETON FAMILY 1895-1913

Not long after the family built their new home and became settled on Farwell Avenue, they sent for Grandmother Adaline Larimore, Jessie's mother in Minneapolis, to come and live with them. Grandmother Larimore also had a passion for botanical things; her fondness was for flowers. She came by train, carrying several pots of geraniums in order to establish "a bit of color" on the frontier. She was astonished upon her arrival in

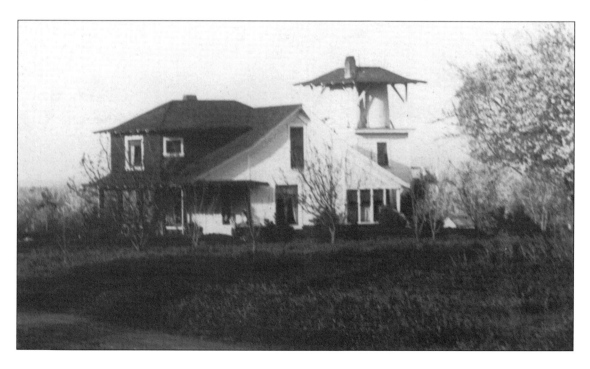

Saratoga to find the temperate climate and beautiful gardens blooming year around. She promptly threw geraniums she had nursed all the way from Minnesota out the train window. Grandmother Larimore became a permanent part of the Pendleton household until her death at age 95.

Two more children were born to Louis and Jessie during their years in Saratoga: Morris Blanchard (b. Feb. 4, 1901; d. Feb. 18, 1985), and David Andrew (b. Aug. 21, 1909; d. 1914).

The family kept several animals on the ranch, a horse named "Pet," an old cow named

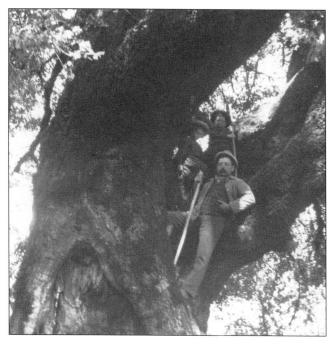

Robert, Lois and Father in giant live oak tree at "Minnewawa" in Santa Cruz mountains above Saratoga, May 1901.
Below: Prune orchard in bloom surrounding Pendleton home on Farwell Avenue, 1903.

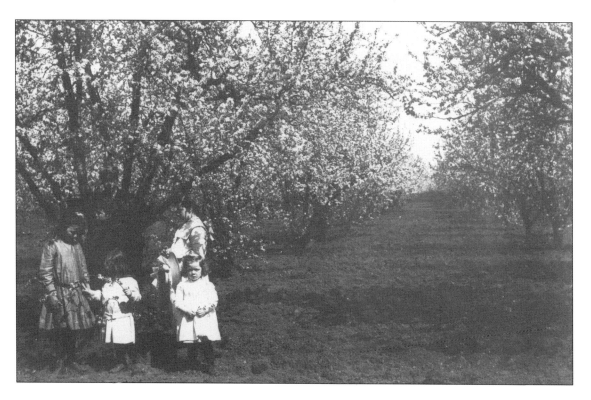

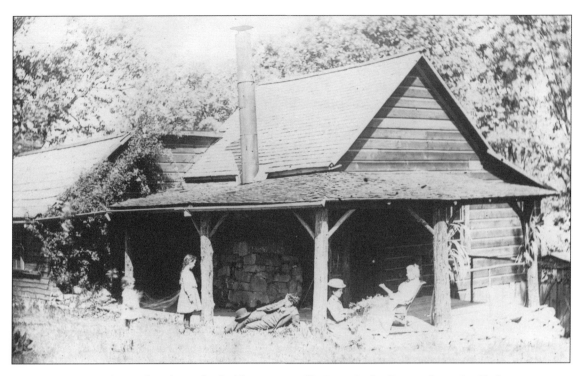

Pendleton family at the "Old Homestead", Deer Ridge Farm along the Skyline in Santa Cruz mountains, 1903.
Below: Pendleton family enjoy their vacations at the "Old Homestead".

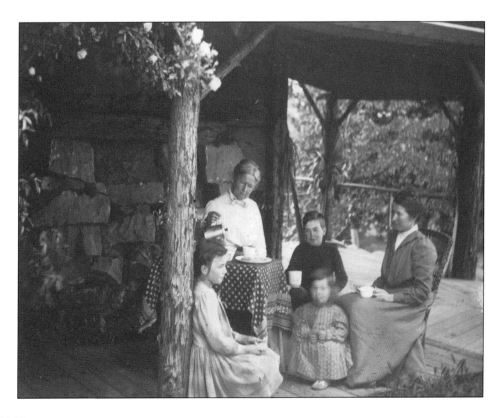

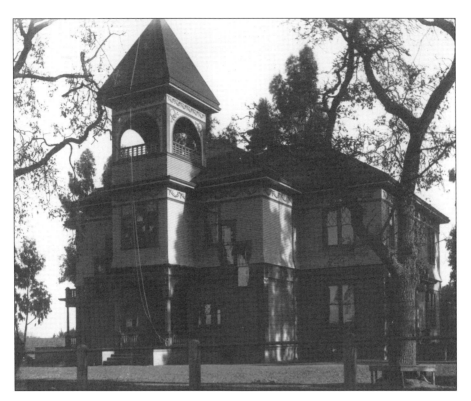

"Daisy" who provided milk for the family, chickens in a chicken yard, and by 1899 a pet donkey named "Topsy" for the children to ride.

Saratoga Grammar School about 1904.
Below: Saratoga Congregational Church about 1904.

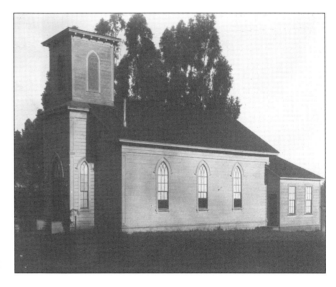

Farwell Glen, on the Bella Vista estate, was directly across Farwell Avenue from the Pendleton home and a favorite place for the children and their friends to play. There were meadows of buttercups and forget-me-nots, big trees to climb, brooks and streams for sailing boats, Wild-Cat Creek, where they went fishing near Ah Hoo's cabin, natural bridges crossing the brooks, and thickets and glens to explore. Ah Hoo was the Farwell's caretaker on their extensive estate, Bella Vista.

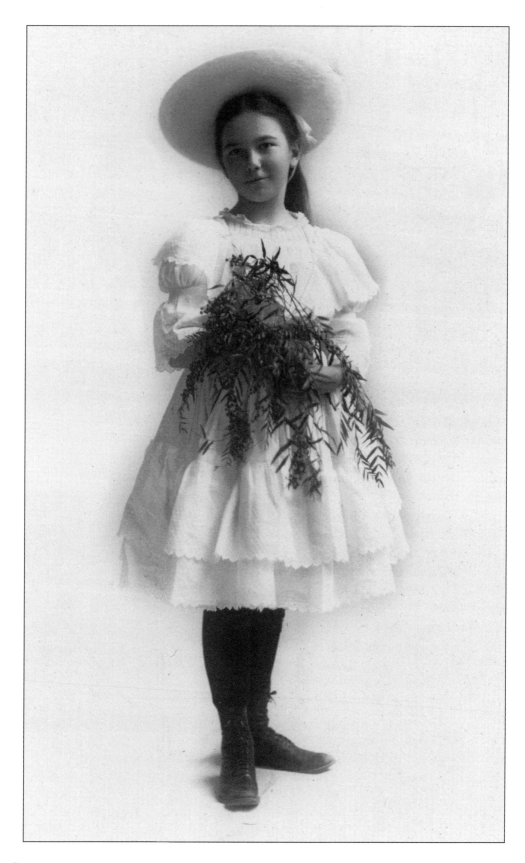

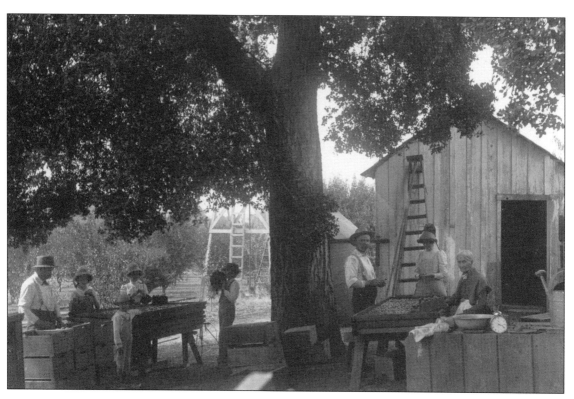

Cutting apricots at Mills-Waterhouse place, 1905.
Left: Lois Pendleton age 10, Jan. 1905.
Right: "P. P. P. P." Pendleton's Prize Prune Pickers
Morris, Father and Lois
with padded knees.

Jessie, a school teacher in Minnesota before her marriage, directed her activities toward music and education. The way she tutored Robert, Lois, and Morris made their grammar school years easy and they excelled in school. Educational encouragement came from two directions, their teachers in the Saratoga Grammar School and their mother's tutoring.

During their childhood on the ten acre prune

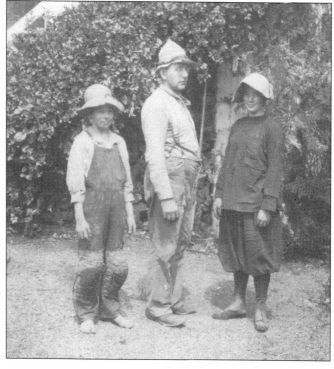

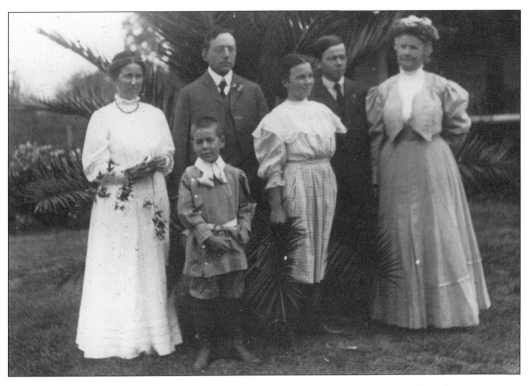

Pendleton family in 1906: Mother, Morris, Father, Lois, Robert and Grandmother Larimore.

ranch, the trees were young and starting to bear, so the children were pressed into picking the prune crop every August and September. The children were paid 4 cents for each 40 pound box. They supplemented this income by working for neighbors as well. Prunes when ripe drop to the ground and are gathered on hands and knees. Their mother sewed thick knee pads into their overalls so they could scramble around on the ground without hurting themselves. The family was known as the P.P.P.P.'s, or the Four P's, (Pendleton's Prize Prune Pickers).

SAN FRANCISCO EARTHQUAKE IN 1906

When the famous San Francisco earthquake occurred in April 1906, Lois was twelve years old and sleeping in the bedroom her father had built for her under the water tower or "tank house" behind their home. She awakened to a rocking motion with water sloshing around in her bedroom and wondered if a tidal wave had come across the Santa Cruz mountains. She waded to her bedroom window which faced north toward San Francisco and the sky was red with the flames of San Francisco burning to the ground. She didn't know whether she was awake or having a nightmare!

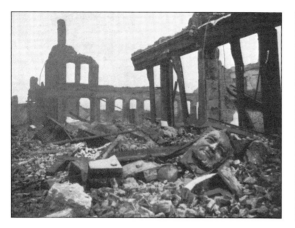
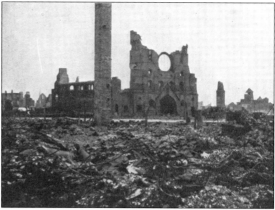

Robert, her older brother, was fascinated by the effects of the earthquake and took many photographs of orchard trees moved out of line by the slippage along the San Andreas fault, which ran from San Francisco through Saratoga. Roads moved out of line and a front porch slipped sideways along the front of a house; vertical drops also occurred in a few places (such as Paul Masson vineyard). Robert was so interested in the effects of the earthquake that he decided to study geology at the university.

San Francisco earthquake, April 1906

CAMPBELL UNION HIGH SCHOOL

Lois and Robert attended Campbell Union High School, the nearest high school with full college preparatory curriculum. It was located eight miles east from Saratoga. Robert rode his bicycle to and from Campbell Union High School five days a week, and Lois rode her horse the sixteen mile round-trip each day. As a child she longed to have her own horse and worked toward that goal by picking prunes year after year and saving her money. Finally, when she was ready to start high school, she had saved enough to buy herself a horse,

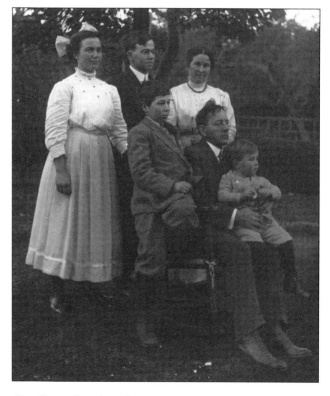

Pendleton family, Christmas 1912: Lois age 18, Robert, Morris, Mother, Father and David.

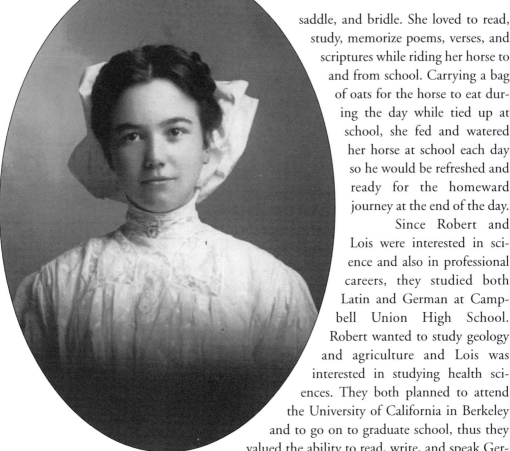

Lois age 16 in 1910.

saddle, and bridle. She loved to read, study, memorize poems, verses, and scriptures while riding her horse to and from school. Carrying a bag of oats for the horse to eat during the day while tied up at school, she fed and watered her horse at school each day so he would be refreshed and ready for the homeward journey at the end of the day.

Since Robert and Lois were interested in science and also in professional careers, they studied both Latin and German at Campbell Union High School. Robert wanted to study geology and agriculture and Lois was interested in studying health sciences. They both planned to attend the University of California in Berkeley and to go on to graduate school, thus they valued the ability to read, write, and speak German. This annoyed their younger brother Morris because, when Lois and Robert wanted to talk about something that interested them and prevent Morris from understanding their conversation, they would talk in German.

Active in athletics during her high school years, Lois played on the girls' basketball team at Campbell High School. When Father heard on his travels about the new game called tennis, he obtained information about rules and dimensions of the court and built a clay tennis court in their prune orchard next to the family home on Farwell Avenue. Lois learned to play tennis as a youngster and became very skilled at the sport, winning many singles and doubles tournaments in high school and college, also later while living in north China. Tennis was her favorite athletic activity, which she enjoyed playing into her sixties.

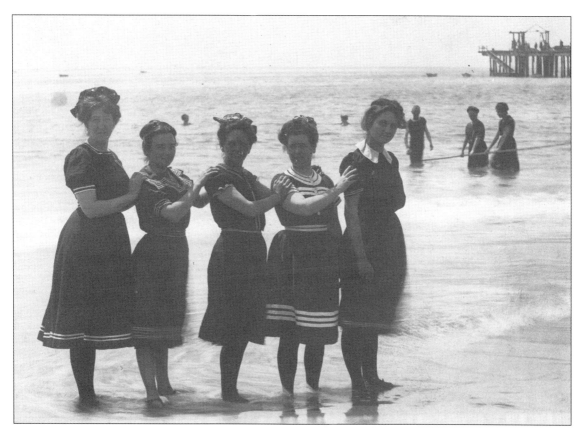

FOOTHILL STUDY CLUB

Jessie, their mother, was a charter member of the Foothill Study Club, organized by several neighborhood women over sewing and teacups in the home of Miss Lyra Mills on Jan. 22, 1907. Their inspiration came from Mrs. George Waterhouse who was living in far away Ketchikan, Alaska. She had become involved with a small, informal study group and had found it so stimulating she proposed a similar one to her sister, Miss Lyra Mills, in Saratoga, her home town. The twelve charter members were: Miss Lyra Mills, Miss Ethel Foster, Mrs. Frances

Bathing beauties ready to swim at beach in Santa Cruz. (Lois second from left.)
Lois and her friend Icile Wilson in a fishing boat at Santa Cruz.

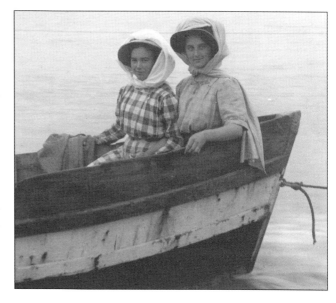

Williams (wife of the Rev. "Sunshine" Williams), Mrs. Adele Richards, Miss Laura Richards, Mrs. Helen Plant, Miss Florence Stone, Mrs. E. A. Norton, Miss Jennie Farwell, Mrs. J. L. Pendleton, Mrs. George Foster, and Mrs. F. W. Mills.

Although it was an informal group, their study plans were ambitious. They launched their first project with "The Cities of the Mediterranean" and within a short time the members were deep in researching ancient history and archaeology. In addition, they were also interested in community betterment. Although the organization was simple, they embarked on challenging subjects. From the beginning, they invited well traveled, talented women with artistic and literary ability to share their experiences with members who were eager for further advancement. Meetings were well attended and members were assigned to do research and give reports on various subjects.

FAMILY OF JOHN BROWN OF HARPER'S FERRY

Jessie's friends in Saratoga included Sarah Brown, daughter of abolitionist John Brown of Harper's Ferry. Mary Ann Day Brown, widow of John Brown, came to live in Saratoga sixteen years after the Civil War ended. Her two daughters, Sarah and Ellen, and Ellen's husband and three daughters came with her.

Consternation and resentment echoed through the community because local Southerners blamed John Brown with his consuming hatred of slavery as the instigator of the Civil War. Now his widow and her family were to become part of this peaceful community! Mrs. Mary Brown (1816-1884) lived in Saratoga from 1881 to 1883 and was buried in Madronia Cemetery. Sarah Brown worked as an assistant weigher at the U. S. Mint in San Francisco for a brief time. After her mother's death she returned to Saratoga and became an artist and an outstanding citizen, giving unselfishly of her time to all community activities until her death in 1916. Sarah Brown gave Jessie Pendleton one of her still-life pictures, a "Basket of Apples", done in pastel. This picture occupied an honored spot in the Pendleton home. (It now belongs to David Satterthwaite, the son of Jessie's youngest child, Adaline.)

EDUCATIONAL ENRICHMENT

Saratoga was on the annual Chautauqua circuit, offering two or three days of lectures and various special programs. Lois was eager for all manner of information, local, regional and what was commonly referred to in church groups as "the foreign field." The lectures given by missionaries who had served

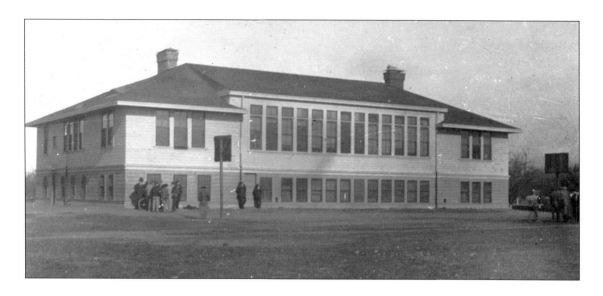

Back of Campbell Union High School about 1908.
Below: Campbell Union High School Basket Ball Team. (Lois at right end.)

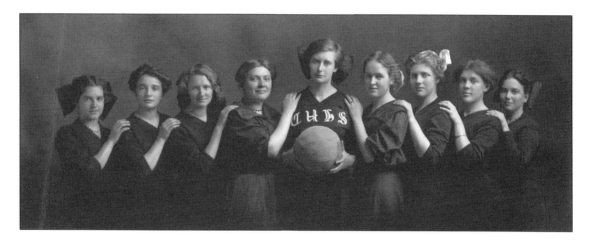

as educators, nurses, and doctors in foreign countries and were home on furlough, fascinated Lois.

The Saratoga school system became less challenging because Robert, Lois, and Morris grew up with a generous supply of periodicals through the mails which supplemented their San Jose newspaper and added depth to their schooling. Both Robert and Lois were avid readers, never realizing at that time how their extensive reading prepared them for their future lives abroad.

Morris's interest in business became evident early. At the age of twelve he established a franchise selling "Success" magazine subscriptions in the farming neighborhood near his family's prune ranch, riding his bicycle from ranch to ranch.

MISSIONARY SETTLEMENT

"The Saratoga Congregational Church from its earliest days had always been an enthusiastic supporter of missionary work," states the book *Saratoga's First Hundred Years,* published by the Saratoga Historical Foundation. Rev. Edwin S. "Eternal Sunshine" Williams (1837-1918), a retired Congregational minister and a man of many ideas, purchased part of the Bella Vista Ranch in 1895. It included the pride of the Farwell family, The Knoll, with its fine oaks and extensive views of both valley and mountains. Sunshine Williams proposed establishing a Missionary Settlement in Saratoga, but his ambitious plans for the Bella Vista Ranch site were too expensive to become a reality. However on April 22, 1900 the Saratoga Missionary Settlement was organized with its object to give counsel, comfort, or assistance to returned missionaries. Officers were President, Rev. W. W. Scudder of Alameda; Vice-Presidents, Rev. H. M. Tenney of San Jose, and Rev. H. W. Cross of Saratoga; Recording Secretary, J. L. Pendleton; Corresponding Secretary, Rev. Edwin S. Williams; Treasurer, Frank M. Farwell; Custodian, Miss Jennie M. Farwell, all of Saratoga.

Search for a site for the Missionary Settlement began at once. After three years, the lots between the church and the parsonage were purchased with special funds collected in Sunday morning church service.

The Settlement members were not the type to wait until they could do big things, so they rented a little cottage on Oak Street. They furnished it comfortably for Rev. Cole, whose health had been seriously impaired by his missionary labors on Douglas Island, Alaska.

In spite of all the zeal and self-sacrifice of the members, the Missionary Settlement never developed as planned. But for many years the same type of service rendered the Coles was given to furloughed missionaries in the attractive home which the Settlement purchased in 1907, at the corner of Oak and St. Charles Streets. While recuperating there, the visiting missionaries became helpful members of the church and community. These missionaries included the Martins from Turkey and Miss Douglas from Sophia, Bulgaria. Their presence, and stories of their experiences and adventures, broadened the horizons of the children and young people of the Congregational Church, inspiring some of them, including Robert and Lois Pendleton, to become missionaries themselves.

COMMUNITY

Saratoga's Blossom Festival was conceived in the spring of 1899, by Rev. Sunshine Williams, as a community celebration of thanksgiving following the welcome end of two years of disastrous California drought. The festival would take place in spring, when the fruit trees of the valley were in bloom, to express

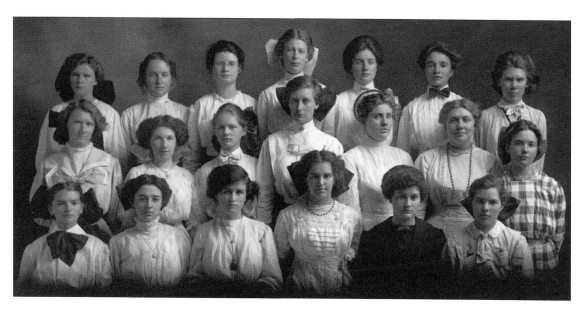

Campbell Union High School Philosophia about 1910. (Lois in plaid dress.)

thankfulness for the harvest to come. He said, "Wouldn't it be a splendid thing if the folks in the cities could see this God-given glory of springtime?" Neighborliness was a way of life for him. So he said, "Why not have a large, old-fashioned country picnic?" Everyone could enjoy not only the snowy blossoms mantling the valley, but other scenic beauties of Saratoga, as well as the friendly hospitality of its people.

Sunshine's unquenchable enthusiasm and boundless energy proved contagious. Within a short time local folk were working on committees for the first Blossom Festival which was held on March 20, 1900. Saratogans drove their wagons to Los Gatos to meet the train and bring the thousands of visitors to Saratoga for scenic tours, a parade, picnic, and concert. The Blossom Festival became a major annual event on a Sunday in March or April when the fruit blossoms reached their peak and the valley was fragrant with the fruit orchards in bloom.

Only a few telephones existed when the Pendleton family arrived in Saratoga in 1895. As telephones became more available, the typical crank-operated telephones had about eight families on each line. When the telephone rang, most of the families would lift the receiver to see if bad news was reported. A farm animal may have broken out of a pasture, a fire or serious illness may have occurred. Consequently, everybody near the area of the subscriber received the message. It was farm communication in its most effective form.

The postman out of Saratoga, who covered his territory with a horse and buggy, provided limited delivery service. When the boys in the neighborhood wanted to know what went on and where, they would follow the postman on their bicycles and read the postal cards in the mail boxes along the road. Lois always reprimanded Morris and his friends for violation of privacy. The boys countered with the argument that if the writer did not want the community to be informed, they would send a sealed letter for 2 cents rather than a postal card for 1 cent.

John Louis Pendleton derived his principal income from traveling as hardware salesman in his extensive territory west of Minneapolis, including Omaha, Kansas City, El Paso, Denver, Salt Lake City, and Spokane. He made three two-month trips by railroad each year. The development of the West was intriguing to many of his business friends and customers east of his territory, so they and a few relatives often visited the Pendleton home in Saratoga. Their stories fascinated Morris and helped to inform the older children, Robert and Lois.

THE MOUNTAIN PLACE, MINNEWAWA

Often Louis and Jessie would hitch up the springwagon and horse and take guests for a ride over the 27 mile drive starting from Saratoga, west up the canyon past Congress Springs, to the summit on the Big Basin road. They turned south along the ridge of the Santa Cruz mountains, with a view of the Pacific ocean and Santa Cruz Bay to the west and a view of Santa Clara Valley to the east, continued down to Los Gatos, and back to Saratoga. The dirt roads were poor with no gravel or asphalt, so the youngsters and men walked along with the horse to make the load easier as they climbed into the mountains. The road along the summit or ridge of the Santa Cruz mountains later came to be known as Skyline Drive.

During these frequent mountain drives Louis would stop the wagon for the children to climb up ladders to the caves of Castle Rock, to enjoy the view, or to admire an unusually large, beautiful tree. One day as he was driving along the ridge he saw a young man with an ax trying to cut down a huge fir tree. Louis stopped the family springwagon and got out to ask the young man why he was cutting down the tree. He wanted to persuade him to spare that handsome, big fir tree. The young man, Fred Herring, explained that he made a living by cutting down trees and selling the wood for lumber. When Louis Pendleton asked Fred Herring how much money he expected to get for the wood, his reply was greeted with an offer from Louis to pay him that sum of money in order to save the tree and buy the ground on which it stood.

This was the first of several land purchases made by Louis along the ridge from Fred Herring and others. Fred and his wife, Lella, became fast friends

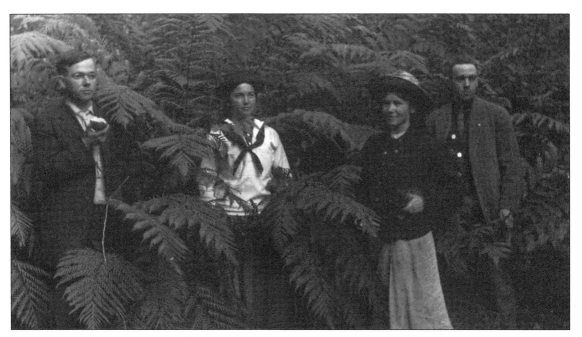

Robert, Lois and friends in Redwood Gulch above Saratoga in the Santa Cruz mountains, Santa Clara County.

of the Pendletons and graciously became caretakers of the pear and apple orchards planted on some of the Pendleton family's Skyline acreage.

Over the years the Pendletons purchased about 150 acres along the ridge of the Santa Cruz mountains, about half on the Santa Cruz side and half on the Santa Clara side.

A beautiful grove of towering redwood trees, along the canyon just above Saratoga on the Santa Clara side, was among the Pendleton family's favorite land acquisitions. They named this acreage "Redwood Gulch." Its lush ferns, wildflowers and birds, became Lois's favorite retreat. She and Robert and friends would hike up the canyon from Saratoga for picnics and other outings in the redwoods.

On one occasion that Morris could never forget, the family party started from home with a picnic lunch for a mountain outing by horse and spring-wagon. They had promised Morris that he could go along. His assignment before departure was to place Saturday's and Sunday's supply of wood in the big wood box by the kitchen stove. Morris was all ready to go with clean overalls on and as he started to climb into the springwagon, his father asked him if he had completed his chore. Morris sheepishly admitted he had not. His father said "Sorry, Morris" and spoke to the horse and off they went without him. Grandmother Larimore, who always took the part of the youngsters, said "Let's hurry and fill the wood boxes and intercept them." So they both fell to and completed the job. They climbed into the buggy, harnessed up another horse and set off at a gallop, intercepting them just before they started up the first hill. Father asked if Morris had completed his assignment and, when he said enthusiastically that he had, with the help of Grandmother, Father said "Get aboard". The subject was closed.

Lois, who was already in the springwagon, immensely enjoyed this brief chain of events which was a lifelong lesson to her on parental discipline and youthful compliance. Robert stayed home that day and worked on his extensive stamp collection, at which he excelled.

Their father, Louis, spent as much as two months at home between sales trips. If farm work eased up, the family of five would go to a cabin at Deer Ridge, on the summit of the Castle Rock ridge, for a few weeks and Morris would walk three miles to a one room schoolhouse. Morris liked the easy sociability with the youngsters and enjoyed the fiendish pleasure of trying boyhood irritations on a new teacher. Lois, in high school by then, often found reading and studying at home with Grandmother preferable.

Father, a county road commissioner, frequently traveled the roads in the area and recommended new routes for other roads. Father managed to squeeze time from his work as prune rancher and traveling salesman to be county road commissioner and to serve in many other civic activities. He enjoyed responsibility and being involved with decision making; he was eager to participate in worthwhile causes.

The Pendletons referred to their mountain property as the Mountain Place or "Minnewawa" (from Longfellow's poem "Song of Hiawatha"), the Indian word for the murmur of wind in the trees. The Herring property was known as Deer Ridge Farm. The family often stayed with Fred and Lella Herring at Deer Ridge Farm or down in the Spring Cabin in their mountain fruit orchard. The family always made trips to Minnewawa in September to pick pears and apples. They put the fruit in lug boxes to carry home and Mother and Grandmother canned many quarts for the winter.

Other outings the family enjoyed tremendously were trips to the seashore via Los Gatos to Capitola, Santa Cruz, and Pacific Grove, where the family would rent a cottage. They loved exploring the Seventeen Mile drive south of Monterey to Carmel and Point Lobos, a spectacular rocky prominence south of Carmel, which was a favorite because of rocks to climb and tide pools to explore.

Jessie, was very musical, had a lovely contralto voice, and played the piano. She sang in the Congregational Church choir and played the piano for the church in Saratoga. Lois began to study the piano as soon as the family was able to purchase one, becoming an advanced pianist by the time she was in high school. She also enjoyed singing in the church and school choirs. She too had a lovely voice, singing both soprano and alto. During her university years she played the Spanish guitar, which went to China with her after she completed her medical training.

Lois placed heavy educational emphasis on sciences as she hoped to become a public health nurse or physician and work as a medical missionary in a foreign land. She graduated with honors from Campbell Union High School in 1912 and entered University of California in Berkeley that Fall.

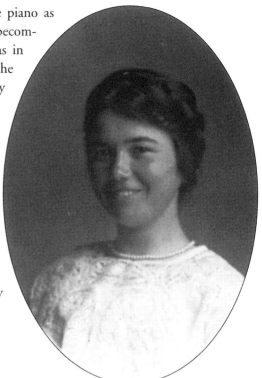

Lois age 18 in 1912, high school graduation picture.

CHAPTER 3

Berkeley Student Years

Lois enrolled in the College of Arts and Sciences at University of California in Berkeley in September 1912. She and Robert rented a cottage at 2219 Dwight Way, Berkeley, their home for the academic year. In July 1913 the Pendleton family sold the prune ranch in Saratoga and moved to a small bungalow at 2342 Eunice Street, high in the Berkeley hills, about one mile uphill from the Univer-

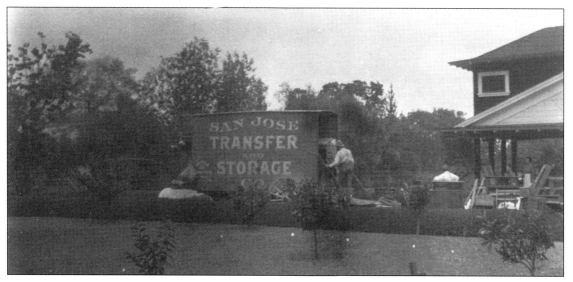

Pendleton family moving from Saratoga to Berkeley, July 1913.

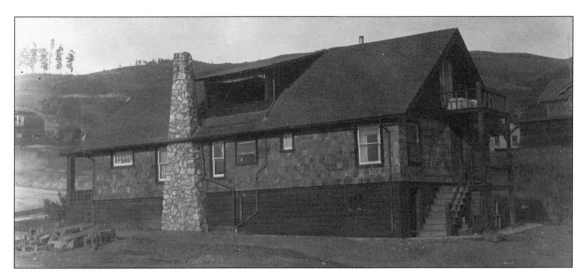

sity of California campus. Father sold his fruit growing properties in Saratoga and moved the family to Berkeley on July 24, 1913 in

Bungalow purchased by Pendleton family on Eunice Street in Berkeley hills.

order to provide a home environment for Robert and Lois during their university years.

The property Father bought on Eunice street had a one and a half story bungalow. Though too small for the family, it was conveniently located close to the campus and was served by the Euclid Electric Street Car Line; the trolley car traveled up the hills and stopped at Eunice Street. Cordonices Park, an extensive park with hills and valleys that gave the Pendleton family the feeling they were still in the country, was along the back of the property. It also had a panoramic view of San Francisco Bay, Golden Gate, and Mount Tamalpais.

Soon after arriving in Berkeley, Father had the bungalow jacked up and the foundation removed, the building raised enough to put a full story underneath, and the attic enlarged to a full story above, converting the bungalow to a three story home with panoramic views and ample place for a library and bedrooms for Robert, Lois, and Morris on the top floor. During the construction period the family lived in two canvas tents next to the house. It was summer so camping was no problem weatherwise.

The Pendleton property backed up to a gulley spanned by a long, high trestle. The family's penchant for gardening resulted in a 100 foot row of artichokes inside their garden wall. On the Eunice Street frontage Father built a lattice fence along which he planted Cecil Bruner roses. Whenever Father left the house, Mother placed a Cecil Bruner rosebud in the button hole of his suit coat.

In those days Father was driving a 1909 Carter Car. The Carter had a friction drive, same as the Saxon car, the only two makes of cars which had a friction drive; Father was enamored with this because he had started a small shop in

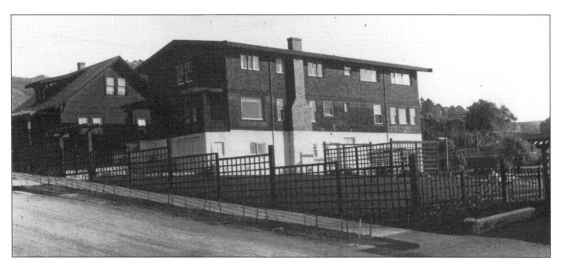

Bungalow converted to three story home, street view.
Below: Bungalow converted to three story home, rear view with tennis court.

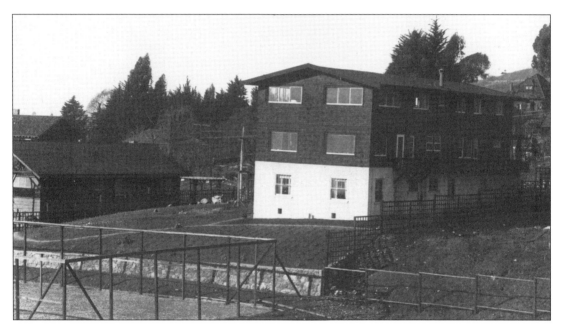

San Jose in 1901-1902 making automobiles with a friction drive. He gave up on this business soon after it started because his partner was a tool maker at heart. Each of the five to six models were "tool room jobs," each one including mechanical advantages not in the previous model. Because Father's partner could not comprehend the principle of sticking with a model once developed and going into mass production, Father gave up the operation. Next the family transportation changed to a secondhand 1914 Cadillac touring car, which the family kept until about 1928.

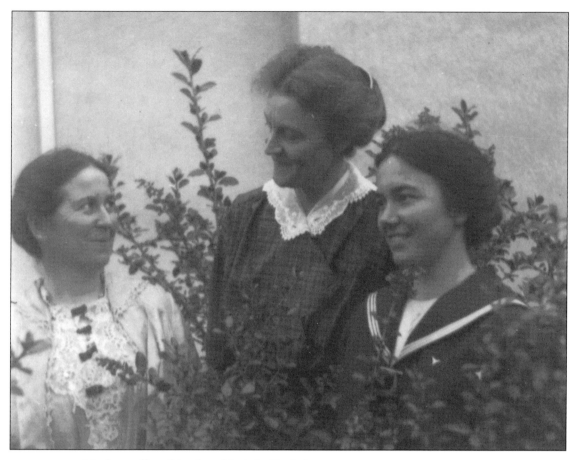

Mother, college friend and Lois in Berkeley.
Below: Clark Waterhouse, childhood friend and neighbor, killed in World War I.

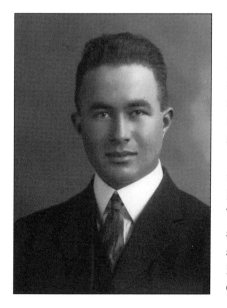

In 1914 David was old enough to go to a Berkeley Public School kindergarten. He contracted diphtheria there and died in December 1914 at the age of five. There were 32 positive throat cultures in the kindergarten. The Pendletons were grief stricken at the loss of their little son.

By 1914 World War I had started, dominating the economy and all public activities. The war did not interfere with Lois's and Robert's long-range plans. They continued to prepare for careers in medicine and agriculture respectively. Clark Waterhouse, neighbor and childhood playmate of Lois in Saratoga, died serving as a soldier in World War I. Lois grieved over Clark's death as she had hoped to marry him someday.

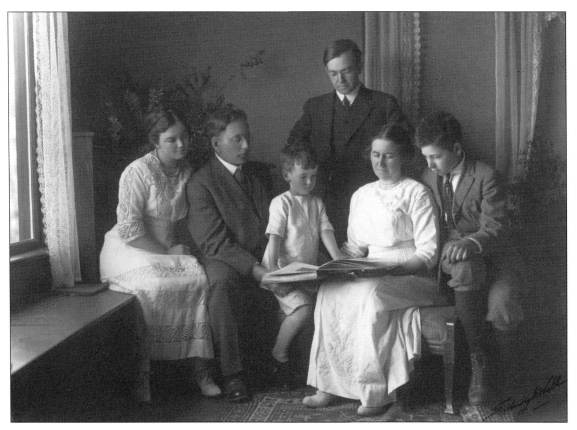

The Silver Wedding Anniversary, June 24, 1914 - in library of Pendleton home in Berkeley: Lois, Father, David, Robert, Mother and Morris.

Morris attended junior high and high school in Berkeley, graduating in 1918 from Berkeley High School. Father was already in Los Angeles, having become a partner in the Plomb Tool Company. He purchased a house on Kingsley Drive, on the near west side of the fast growing metropolitan Los Angeles area.

With Morris accepted by Pomona College's wartime student army training corps, Lois deep in her medical studies at the University of California School of Medicine in San Francisco, and Robert teaching abroad in India, the Pendleton family moved from Berkeley to southern California.

Robert received a B.S. in Agriculture in 1914 and Ph.D. in Agriculture in 1917. After graduation he married Anne Miltimore from Corvallis, Oregon, who had spent her high school years near Saratoga. Their paths crossed again later when she was teaching school in Riverside. Anne lost her hearing during her college years in Los Angeles when she contracted typhoid fever while attending Normal School (teacher's college). While Anne taught school in Ripon, California she boarded with Aunt Jennie Lawton, sister of Jessie Larimore Pendleton. Robert and Anne were married June 10, 1917 before sailing for the Orient where

Robert had a teaching position awaiting him at the Presbyterian mission College of Agriculture in India.

Both Robert and Lois earned honors at the University of California at Berkeley and were involved with Y.M.C.A. and Y.W.C.A., Cosmopolitan Club, and Student Volunteers.

Adaline was born in Berkeley on Feb. 7, 1917 and named for her Grandmother Adaline Larimore who was born Feb. 11, 1839, seventy-eight years earlier. The arrival of the new baby helped to fill the empty space left by little David's death. Adaline was 23 years younger than her sister Lois and 27 years younger than her brother Robert.

During the Berkeley years, Louis had continued his work as traveling hardware salesman. On one of his trips through the Pacific Northwest in December 1916, he was spending the night at the Davenport Hotel in Spokane, Washington. He met a "fellow Gideon" named Charles H. Williams in the hotel lobby. They struck up a conversation and found they had many common interests.

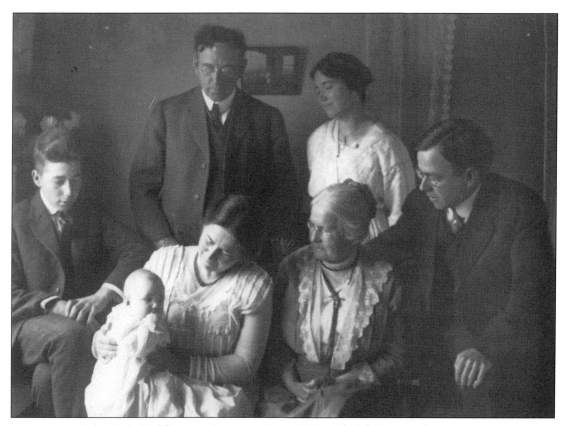

The 28th Wedding Anniversary, June 1917 with Adaline age four months.

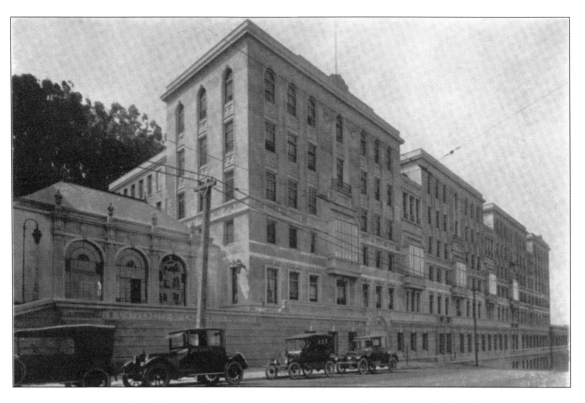

University of California Hospital in San Francisco, where Lois studied medicine 1916–1920.
Below: Lois in 1919 with her baby sister, Adaline, 23 years younger.

During their conversation Mr. Williams received a telegram from the managing director of Plomb Tool, informing him that his partner, Bill Ziegler, had just died from strep throat and that he should hurry home. Mr. Williams turned to Louis and said, "Why don't you join me in the Plomb Tool Company?" Without hesitation, but after careful thought, Louis decided that tool manufacturing, rather than tool sales, would create for him an interesting new challenge and an opportunity for advancement. So they became partners and Louis Pendleton moved to Los Angeles. August Plomb, a skilled tool forger, was making the hand-forged automotive

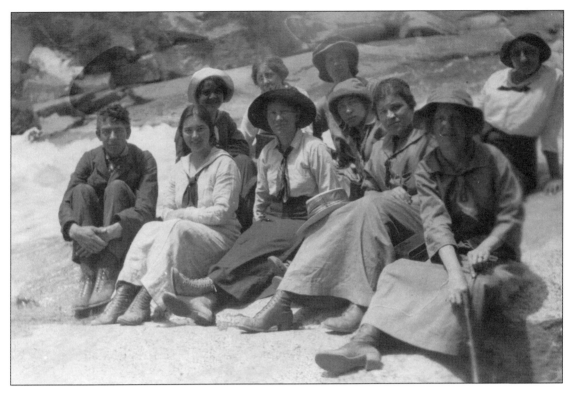

Lois and hiking friends at top of Yosemite Falls.
Below: Lois (on right) reading in front of her tent at Yosemite, where she
worked for Camp Curry Company during college summer.

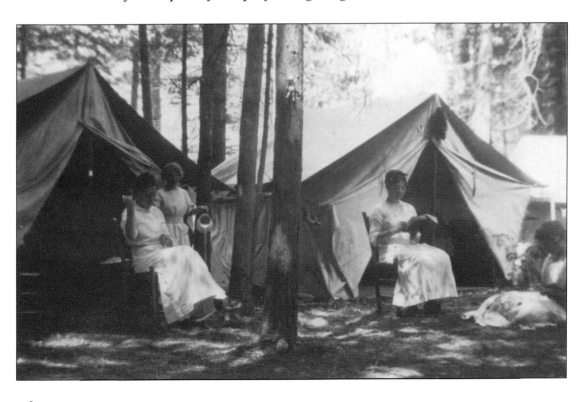

tools since 1907 at the Los Angeles blacksmith shop owned by Charles H. Williams and Bill Ziegler.

Lois received her A.B. in Arts and Sciences in 1916 and her M.D. in 1920 from the University of California Medical School, after one year of internship at San Francisco City and County Hospital. During college, Lois demonstrated the high energy and drive that characterized her adult years. In addition to academic honors, she taught Sunday School, played the Spanish guitar, sang, and continued to study piano. She played tennis frequently on the tennis court her father built next to their home on Eunice Street.

She enjoyed wonderful work experiences and hiking in Yosemite National Park and Grand Canyon National Park during the summers of her university years. She was strong, athletic, and energetic. She loved challenge and adventure. During her undergraduate years she spent a summer working for the Curry Park Company as a summer employee at Ahwanee Lodge, Yosemite. This experience gave her the opportunity to enjoy this magnificent park with lots of hiking and climbing with her colleagues, and also to save money for school.

Lois while in medical school in San Francisco.

She spent another summer during her under-graduate years working at Grand Canyon. Her strength and stamina were amazing. One day, starting before dawn, she hiked to the bottom of Grand Canyon and back up to the rim all in one day. To do the round-trip by foot in one day was a remarkable feat. It required jogging a good part of the way, as well as dodging other hikers, donkeys and pack-mules.

On Sept. 1, 1920 Lois and her medical school classmate, Dr. Alma Cooke, were commissioned by the American Board of Commissioners for Foreign Missions (Congregational Church) to serve as physicians in China. The commissioning service took place as part of the 47th annual meeting of the Woman's Board of Missions for the Pacific, held at the First Congregational Church in Oakland, California. Hymns included "O, Master Let Me Walk With Thee" and "From Greenland's Icy Mountains." Following their commissioning,

Dr. Lois Pendleton and Dr. Alma Cooke sailed for their separate posts as physicians in Shantung province, China.

The Pendleton family continued to keep their mountain acreage, Minnewawa, in the Santa Cruz mountains above Saratoga for pleasure and for future retirement. Each September they returned to their mountain fruit orchard, picking pears and apples for fresh eating and canning them for the winter. They also visited the Pendleton family plot in Saratoga's Madronia Cemetery.

While Father and Mother were living in the Sierra Vista area of Los Angeles, they became actively involved in the newly organized Oneonta Congregational Church of South Pasadena, first worshiping in a bungalow and later in a new building on Fletcher Avenue, South Pasadena. Morris and his wife, Gladys, also made Oneonta their church during their San Marino years.

In 1921, before Morris graduated from Pomona College in 1922, the family moved to a large two story home on Berkshire Drive in Sierra Vista. The lawn was terraced and Father used to mow it saying that this was his exercise instead of playing golf like his business associates. At meals the family would read and discuss letters from Lois in China and from Robert and Anne in India, and later the Philippines. The family lived in Sierra Vista until 1924 when Father, age 57, died unexpectedly.

Morris had joined the tool manufacturing business two years earlier when he graduated from college; he had worked at Plomb Tool Company during his school vacations throughout college. Upon his graduation, two years before Father's death, he joined the company full time. Father had planned to turn the daily management of the business over to Morris, while he continued his quarterly selling trips to the western states hardware stores and made at least

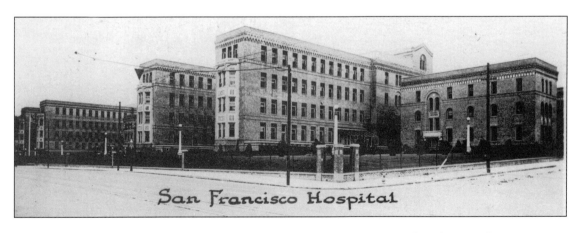

San Francisco Hospital (City and County) where Lois served twelve month rotating internship before receiving her medical degree from University of California in 1920.

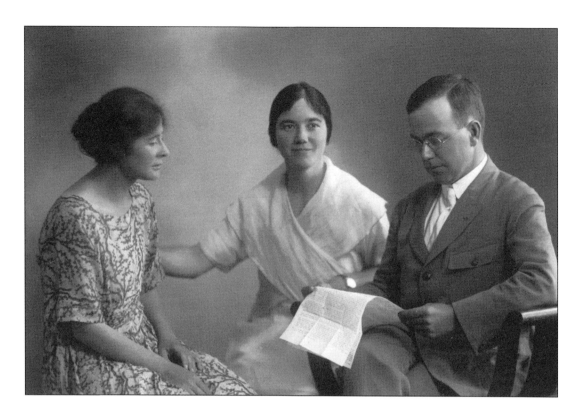

Lois (center) with brother Robert Pendleton and his wife, Anne Miltimore, just before they sailed for India to teach at the Agricultural College.

one trip to Bridgeport, Connecticut, annually to the Stanley Rule and Level Co. Though they discussed Morris's studying for an MBA at Harvard Business School, it was decided instead that Father would take Morris on a trip across country to meet Father's business friends. Morris was working his way up to general manager following this trip when his father died.

While on a business trip to Denver and Salt Lake City in March 1924, Father developed a middle ear infection which led to mastoid infection. He was brought home critically ill and taken directly from the train station to the hospital where he remained for two weeks, finally succumbing to pneumococcal pneumonia on April 7, 1924. Antibiotics were not available at that time.

Morris married his college sweetheart, Gladys Shepard, on August 30, 1924. He became general manager of Plomb Tool Company at a salary of $35 per week. When his father died, Morris invested all his savings, as well as his father's insurance benefits, into the tool manufacturing business. Morris became president of Plomb Tool Company in 1936.

When Father died, Adaline was only seven years old. Changes came quickly. The family home was sold and Mother, Grandmother Larimore, and little Adaline moved to Claremont in the summer of 1925, renting a house on 11th Street. Lois visited her mother and little sister there when she came home on furlough from June 1925 to June 1926. When Lois discovered Mother was still deeply grief-stricken and depressed more than a year after Father's death, Lois decided to take her and little Adaline back to China with her. Lois hoped the change of scenery would help them recover from their grief.

There were insufficient funds to purchase a round trip ticket for Mother, as the proceeds from Father's life insurance had been invested by Morris in the Plomb Tool Company. So Mother, filled with grief, sailed to China on a one way ticket, hoping that funds would become available in a year to purchase a ticket to return home again. A round trip ticket at half-fare was purchased for Adaline at age nine because she would need a full fare ticket at age ten. Mother and Adaline ended up staying in the Orient for nearly two years. Before departing, they arranged for Grandmother Larimore a temporary home with family friends.

When Mother and Adaline returned to California in February 1928, Grandmother Larimore broke her hip and they had to stay in Pasadena while Grandmother was hospitalized in Huntington Memorial Hospital. Mother Pendleton acted as manager for apartments purchased earlier by her husband as an investment. In 1929 Mother rented a house on West 8th Street. Later when Adaline was ready for college, they moved to a home on the Pomona College campus near the power plant (where the Pendleton Women's Athletic Fields are now located) across Second Street from the wildlife preserve, known to generations of students and alumni as the "Wash."

CHAPTER 4

Surgeon in Tehchow

ARRIVAL

In September 1920 Dr. Lois Pendleton and her medical school class-mate, Dr. Alma Cooke, were commissioned by the American Board of Commissioners for Foreign Missions (Congregational Church) to serve as physicians and surgeons in China. Lois was assigned to Williams-Porter Hospitals at the mission station in Tehchow and Alma was assigned to the hospital at the mission station in Lintsing, both in Shantung province.

Lois and Alma sailed for China soon after their commissioning. They met their fellow A.B.C.F.M. missionaries in Hawaii and also in Japan when the ship stopped for a few days to unload and load cargo. After a few months of intense Chinese language school in Peking, Lois and Alma proceeded by train to their hospital stations in Shantung province. Proficiency in the Chinese language was essential to communicating with their patients. It was also vital to the supervision and training of hospital staff, including the training of Chinese nurses. So Lois and Alma continued their study of the Chinese language with private tutors once a week during their years of medical work at Tehchow and Lintsing.

The new recruits were warmly welcomed at their mission stations. The hospitals were understaffed, in serious need of more physicians, especially well trained young physicians with stamina and commitment. The missionaries and their children appreciated the new young physicians with their vigor, enthusiasm, kind dispositions, and good humor. Dr. Lois Pendleton was a special favorite of the children at the Tehchow mission station because of her many athletic interests and her willingness to include the children.

The new doctors discovered relentless demands upon their time. Along with time required for language study, they fulfilled all the usual clinic and hospital duties including handling emergencies, critical patient care, and general surgery. Civil war, bandits, guerrilla skirmishes, floods, famines, and epidemics interrupted their medical responsibilities.

The North China mission of the American Board of Commissioners for Foreign Missions, known as Kung Li Hui, held annual meetings in Peking and interim meetings in the provinces for their missionaries. These gave the young doctors an opportunity to meet with colleagues at other mission stations to share experiences and gain spiritual renewal. Although Tehchow and Lintsing were both located in northwest Shantung province, only 60 miles apart, it was a three day journey by "Peking cart" pulled by donkey over rutted dirt roads, or about 100 miles by boat on the Grand Canal. Visits between Lois and Alma were usually limited to meetings of the Shantung Mission or the North China mission. Telephones had not reached the provinces, existing only in major cities.

GEOGRAPHY

Shantung is a vast flat agricultural plain, south of Tientsin, bisected by the Yellow River (Hwang Ho) which flows from west to east into the Gulf of Chihli (Po Hai). The Grand Canal (Yun Ho), dividing the Shantung plain from north to south, passes through Tehchow. This man-made waterway, constructed during the Ch'in Dynasty (259-210 B.C.) to connect the capital cities of North China with the capital cities of South China, enabled the unification of China by improving commerce between north and south, the movement of army troops, and the collection of taxes. The railroad linking Peking-Tientsin to Tsinan-Suchow-Nanking also passes through Tehchow. The Germans and the French constructed the railroad in the early 1900's.

In 1920 Tehchow, located along the east bank of the Grand Canal in Shantung province, was a small city surrounded by a wall, giving it the appearance of an ancient or medieval city. A railroad station stood outside the west gate of the city. The mission compound was located one third mile east of the city. Tehchow had no rickshaws so everyone walked the one and a half miles from the train station to the mission compound, except Dr. Emma Tucker who rode horseback. The streets of Tehchow were ten to fifteen feet wide with stores and other adobe buildings crowded close together along the streets.

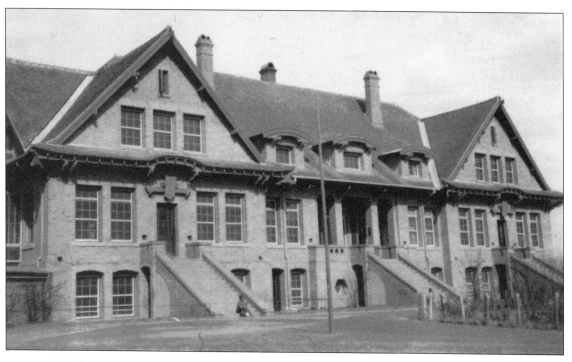

Williams Porter Hospital at Tehchow, Shantung, China where Dr. Lois Pendleton worked as physician and surgeon from 1920 to 1927.

MISSION COMPOUND

 The mission compound, built of two and three story grey brick buildings with grey tile roofs and green shutters, included a boys' school (grades 1-12); a girls' school (grades 1-12); classroom buildings and dormitories; administration building-dispensary and two hospitals (one for men and one for women and children); dining hall; and residences for the staff. A grey brick wall and a dike surrounded the entire compound.

 Tehchow is famous for the high quality bricks made locally. The Ming Emperor selected them for the construction of the Imperial Palace, the Forbidden City, in Peking in 1420 A.D. The Grand Canal was used to transport these bricks on barges from Tehchow to Peking.

 In March and April of 1920, flood threatened the mission. A dike was built around the mission compound by several hundred men who worked for weeks to protect the compound from the possibility of another serious flood as occurred in 1917. They hauled earth in small Chinese wheel-barrows from nearby places in the compound which later became ponds. When about a foot of dirt was dumped, it was pounded, tamped with a flat stone that had eight ropes attached to it and a man holding each rope. The coolies raised and dropped

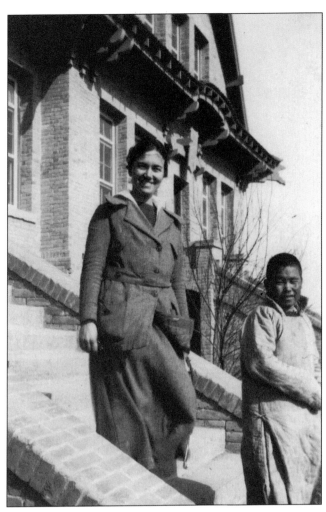

A windy day on hospital steps —Lois with a crippled charity patient.

the stone by alternately moving apart and together while singing a chant to synchronize their rhythm. The laborers worked at building the dike surrounding the entire compound from six in the morning until seven in the evening, taking only a break for a meal at noon. They lived in the compound, sleeping in dug-out shelters, until the dike was completed. The only opening was the main gate to the compound; sandbags were ready nearby to fill in this opening if another flood came and threatened the buildings in the compound.

Flood protection and other mission activities continued under the experienced eyes of leaders such as Dr. Francis Tucker and his wife Dr. Emma Tucker. They first arrived in China as missionary doctors with A.B.C.F.M. in 1915 and planned and supervised the construction of the mission station at Tehchow in 1916 for the Kung Li Hui (North China mission of the American Board of Commissioners for Foreign Missions). Tehchow was selected for the site of this mission station because of its easy access along the Grand Canal and also along the railroad from Peking and Tientsin to Nanking and Shanghai.

Dr. Francis Tucker continued as the medical director of the Williams-Porter Hospitals for many years. The couple's four children were raised at the Tehchow mission compound, educated at North China American School, inter-denominational boarding school at Tungchow (just east of Peking), when they were old enough. All four Tucker children became physicians like their parents.

Miss Alice Reed went to China in 1916 with other former Grinnell College classmates to help establish Grinnell-in-China, the A.B.C.F.M. North China mission station at Tehchow. Alice Reed, a school teacher, served as principal of the Girls' School at the Tehchow mission for many years. She was an A.B.C.F.M. school teacher in China from 1916 to 1948 and later taught in mission schools in Turkey. Alice Reed was Dr. Lois Pendleton's housemate at Tehchow from 1920 to 1927, both living in Grace House (residence for American single ladies on the staff including two teachers, two nurses, one evangelistic worker, and one medical doctor) at the Tehchow mission compound.

Lois in front of Grace House where she lived from 1920 to 1927.

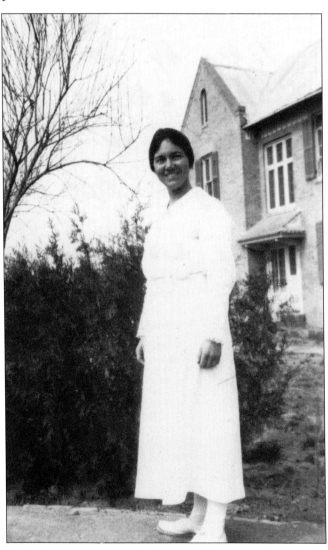

The women divided housekeeping expenses and jobs, including cooking and cleaning. Only thrift could make their salaries of $42 U.S. per month (60 to 80 yuan) plus 46 yuan per month board and room cover their living expenses. Salaries for all were the same, whether one had spent years in medical training, teaching or evangelistic work. Meals were served at 7:00 in the morning, 12:30 mid-day, and 7:00 in the evening.

The compound homes were pleasant; the buildings were constructed of locally made grey brick in a modified Chinese architecture. These houses had no water under pressure. All water for baths had to be carried from the cistern in the basement to the bathroom on the second floor. So one learned to use water sparingly. Rain water was col-

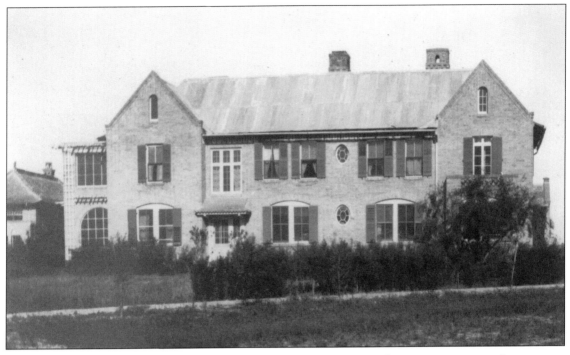

Grace House, residence for single women and guests at the mission compound in Tehchow. Bedroom of Lois under gable at right with French windows.

lected and stored in cisterns underground, as well-water was very alkaline. All drinking water and water for tooth-brushing had to be boiled. Electric lights operated when the old electric generating plant at the mission compound was working, but when it broke down kerosene lamps provided light.

One of the teachers enjoyed gardening, so flowering plants such as geraniums and Angel wing begonias bloomed in the windows and on the porch. Native trees included willow and locust trees. Because of the severe climate, alkaline soil, and frequent drought it was difficult to get other trees to grow. However within the mission compound an effort was made to grow lilacs, hollyhocks, nasturtiums, chrysanthemums, zinnias, vegetables, and even persimmons. Trees were sparse and few.

Dr. Lois Pendleton worked at the hospital from before 7:30 each morning until 6:30 each evening, getting back to the house only for the mid-day meal. She was on duty at the hospital every day and on call every night. She had responsibility for the medical care of all women and children patients, including all surgery.

In 1926 Dr. Lois became excited about the prospect of getting an x-ray machine for the hospital, but a new electric generator had to come first. Electricity to assure lights for the operating room was a higher priority. An x-ray machine was not acquired by the hospital until after Dr. Lois had left Tehchow seven years later.

THE FULL STAFF

The staff at the mission compound in Tehchow in 1920 included Albert (and Clara) Hausske who was superintendent, treasurer, and manager; Dr. Emma Tucker, physician, and Dr. Francis Tucker, physician and medical director, as well as Director of the Red Cross Famine Relief Commission for Shantung; Harold (and Grace) Matthews, pastor; Alfred (and Erma) Heininger, principal of the Boys' School; John Decker, teacher; Alice Reed, principal of the Girls' School; Mabel Huggins, teacher; Helen Dizney, nurse; Myra Sawyer, nurse; and Dr. Lois Pendleton, physician. Dr. Edward (and Marion) Parsons, physician, joined the staff in 1925 and was transferred to the hospital in Tunghsien in 1928. The American staff was supplemented by dedicated Christian Chinese teachers, nurses, and physicians.

RECREATION

Ice skating on the frozen lakes, ponds and on the Grand Canal was a popular winter sport. Dr. Arthur Tucker remembered a cold wintry day in Tehchow in his childhood when Dr. Lois Pendleton came by, ice skates in hand, to inform Arthur and his little brother Frankie that the ice on the pond was thick enough for skating. Sadly, at the time neither of the young Tucker boys had ice skates, so Arthur and Frankie contented themselves with sliding on the ice while Dr. Lois skated around the pond with great gusto. When the Tucker boys reached age ten years, they each went off to boarding school at Tungchow equipped with ice skates and learned to skate and play ice hockey at the North China American School.

Alice Reed remembered a day in January 1925 when she and Lois went skating on the pond in the hospital yard after work. They expected the ice to be thick because of the cold nights, but the water was shallow and the bright midday sun had softened the ice. So it broke and they sank, gradually settling into the knee deep ice-water. But Alice fell twice before she got out, so was well soaked. Fortunately it didn't take the two of them long to get home and into dry clothes.

For exercise at all ages, the missionaries frequently indulged in riding horseback on the local Mongolian ponies. Dr. Lois Pendleton quickly joined the ranks of horse owners, and was very free in making her horse available for the use of any child or adult who knew how to handle reins and bridle. In fact, there were four horse owners in Tehchow mission station at that time, making it possible for all four Tucker children (when the two older ones were home from boarding school) each to have a horse to go on a family outing. Dr. Lois' large white Arabian horse was the most spirited, however, and much more than some persons could handle or dared to ride. The Arabian loved to run like the wind and always won a race.

In 1921 Alice Reed wrote to her family: "I have been horseback riding two or three times and have played tennis once. Dr. Lois Pendleton is a great believer in exercise and insists on others taking exercise. Not a bad thing." When Dr. Lois Pendleton arrived at Tehchow in 1920 she was pleased to find a clay tennis court had been built in the mission compound, and she encouraged the missionaries to play tennis as often as their schedules permitted and to keep fit and enjoy exercise. Tennis was Dr. Lois Pendleton's favorite sport and she played it as often as her busy schedule permitted.

In 1923 Alice Reed wrote: "Friday afternoon I had a horseback ride with Lois and my arm is sore from holding the horse. He was feeling fine and was crazy to race with Lois, of course. I was on the Heininger horse which the Matthews and I are going to buy. We pay only fifteen dollars United States money each, which isn't much for half a horse and a saddle." Lois had taught Alice Reed to ride horseback, and in 1922 when Alice needed to make a country trip to check several schools in the region she asked Lois to go with her on horseback rather than making the journey by donkey cart. They were able to make the round of village schools on horseback in four days, rather than ten days by cart. Mr. Heininger, principal of the Boys' School was horrified at these two daring young women going off alone on horseback with the danger of bandits, robbers, and guerrilla bands. They had a safe and efficient journey and said it was far less tiring than going by cart.

A kindred spirit with the new missionary doctor was John Decker, who was teaching at the Boys' Middle School in Tehchow on assignment from the Grinnell-in-China program. John was a lovable young man, full of fun and always joshing, so he got along well with everyone. John and Lois got into trouble however when they took advantage of some free time on Sunday to play catch with a softball on the road behind the Tucker residence. Beyond the road was the Girls' Middle School and in Dr. Emma Tucker's eyes the exercise was to be condemned for two reasons: in China men and women were never to be seen in activities together; and furthermore, the ball activity was a desecration of the Sabbath, the "day of rest", in full view of the impressionable school girls. Dr. Tucker took no action at the time of the inci-

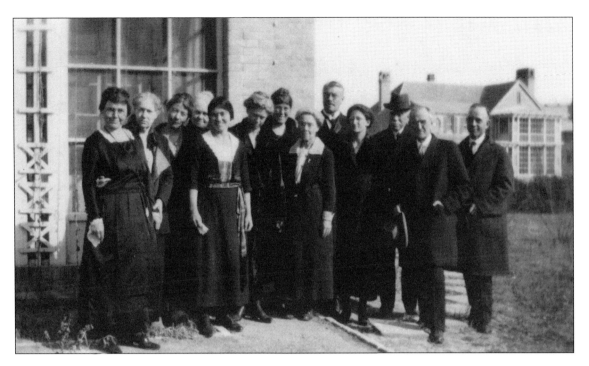

Tehchow mission staff on Thanksgiving 1922: Mabel Huggins (far left) and Lois (front, left of center).

dent, but afterward admonished the two culprits not to ever again undermine the Sabbath.

In 1923 Mabel Huggins and Dr. Lois had an Old Town canoe which they bought second hand in Tientsin and kept in the yard of a Chinese family who lived on the bank of the Grand Canal west of the city of Tehchow. Lois named the canoe "Wawataysee". Mabel Huggins and John Decker took Alice Reed for a ride in the canoe after school. They went by horseback the two miles to the canal, leaving the horses in the same yard where the the boat was kept. They rowed up the canal about a mile and then went ashore for a picnic supper. Dr. Lois and John Decker went horseback riding and canoeing as frequently as her busy schedule permitted. The canoe added a very pleasant variety to their limited recreation. It also afforded recreation on the Sabbath out of the sight of Dr. Emma Tucker.

Flying kites has been a popular sport in China for centuries. One could buy two gorgeous kites for ten cents U.S. money—colorful bats, butterflies, fish, eagles, dragons, and gaily colored ladies. Alice Reed liked to borrow a fishline from Dr. Parsons and have a good time flying the kites in the compound. The kites were made of colorful paper pasted on very light bamboo frames in intricate shapes.

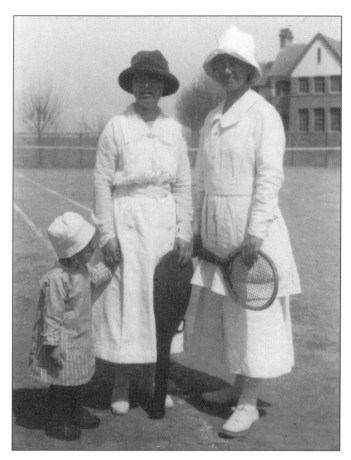

Lois (right) and colleague after a tennis game, Tehchow, Feb. 1923.

DISASTERS

In addition to civil wars between rival war lords, bandit raids and guerrilla skirmishes, dust storms, floods and famines were the major disasters of Shantung province, occurring with regular frequency.

Flood of 1917

In the summer of 1917 a heavy rainy season caused flooding of Tientsin and much of Shantung province along the Grand Canal. By September 23, 1917, the Grand Canal broke its banks, filling the low land between the mission compound and the city of Tehchow and into the mission compound. The men of the staff and servants brought several tons of coal up from the cellar and piled it in bags and barrels on the side porches of the buildings. Everything edible was harvested from the vegetable garden. Flowering plants, ivy, bushes, and small trees were dug up and put into containers on the porches. Every possible vessel was filled with water from the cistern, in anticipation of the dirty polluted flood water contaminating the cistern. About noon the cistern began to fill up with flood water, sounding like Niagara Falls as the flood water rushed in. By the middle of the afternoon it was necessary to build rafts to get from one house to another. Shortly after dinner the mud (adobe) walls which divided the different parts of the compound began to fall, twenty to thirty feet at a time. By the middle of the afternoon the flood water was rising four inches an hour, so the missionaries began moving things from the first floor to the second floor.

When the flood water was three inches deep on the first floor of the buildings, Alice Reed borrowed rubber boots and waded around taking all the doors off their hinges on the first floor and carried them to the second floor. It had been difficult to sleep at night, for all night long there was the the sound of walls and houses outside the compound falling and the swish of water against the houses within the compound. The next morning the water downstairs was too deep for wading and the missionaries began to go out the window at the stairway landing to get onto a raft. That day they evacuated the schoolgirls and sent them to P'angchuang, the former location of the mission station, where church members would take care of the schoolgirls until they could be sent to their homes.

The missionaries decided they should leave their station temporarily as there was no possibility of doing any mission work as long as the flooded condition continued. They got away on October 3, going in small boats to the South Suburb of Tehchow and then walking from there, with men carrying their baggage, on to the Canal, west of the city. Two canal boats had been engaged for the missionaries. The one Alice Reed was in was 9 feet wide and 40 feet long with a cabin 7 feet wide and 20 feet long. When the wind was favorable a square sail was up. Four men rowed with long oars and they had the current with them. When the wind was against them and stronger than the current, the men went ashore and towed the boat. Both boats carried the American flag at the request of the head boatman.

The mission compound at Tehchow was a desolate place when the missionaries left with flood water 32 inches deep on the floors of the buildings and an average of 9 feet deep in the compound. There was a rumor that the Yellow River ("China's Sorrow") had broken into the Grand Canal in several places, thus changing its course.

Because of the breaks in the dikes along the Grand Canal in several places, the water was several feet from the top of the banks. The Canal follows the bed of the Wei River and winds over the flat plain taking 300 miles to make 150 miles to Tientsin. It was lined with trees most of the way and some of them were big and beautiful. The boats tied up at night, traveling only in the day.

Finally they came to a place where the water west of the Canal was higher than the water in the Canal and had broken the banks and was running into the Canal like a great wide river. The boats left the Canal at this point and sailed the rest of the way in to Tientsin over the fields. The flooded area extended to the west and south covering over 150,000 square miles—the worst flood in the area for at least 70 years.

In mid-November one missionary family returned by boat to their station in Tehchow, living only in second floor rooms as the first floor and ground would be in bad shape for some time. Alice Reed and the other Tehchow missionaries returned to their station on December 23, 1917. At the east edge of the city they came to a great sheet of ice; about half a mile across the ice lay their compound. There were three sleds for the little children and the rest walked, carefully avoiding the thin ice where boats had been going back and forth only a few days earlier. The ice was smooth so ice skating was almost limitless, but walking was treacherous.

The missionaries had to bail water out of their cellars for weeks. The thermometer on the north side of the buildings registered 10 to 12 degrees F in the morning and rose to 32 by mid-day. The Tuckers' furnace was started at Thanksgiving and kept going to begin drying things out. The only heat in the classroom building was a small coal stove in the upstairs hall and none in the classrooms. Alice Reed wrote: "I have taken to wearing more clothes -- two woolen union suits, two pairs of stockings (one of them wool), a heavy petticoat, and a wool dress all the time. I got chillblains the first week and my toes swelled up so that I have to wear my gym shoes. I wear gaiters to cover my ankles and put on my rubbers when I go to school. I teach with my big coat on and my hands in my pockets, so that by walking back and forth I keep fairly warm except for my ears."

Dust Storms

Winters in north China are dry, dusty, windy and cold. Temperatures may drop to near zero, with much wind. Snowfall is sparse and infrequent, only a few inches at a time. Lakes remain frozen until March and are popular for ice skating and ice boating.

When Alice Reed went to Tehchow for the dedication of the new church in the South Suburb in early April 1917, a dust storm was in progress when they left Peking. It continued with more or less intensity all the way. "We went through two areas where the air was so thick with dust that one could scarcely see tree trunks against the sky 200 feet away. The sun was completely hidden and the air had a queer yellow look."

Frequent repeated dust storms are common fall, winter and spring in north China, particularly in the month of April. Dust blows in from the Gobi desert far to the northwest across the dry plains, picking up fine yellow topsoil as it moves southeast. The dust storms may occur daily or weekly in the spring and the winds are strong, dry and warm. When a dust storm is on its way the sky suddenly becomes yellow and dark and one can smell the dust and feel the heat of the approaching dust storm. To protect oneself from the choking dust one runs inside, locks windows and doors in haste, closes the eyes, nose, and mouth and holds one's breath or covers the face with a damp handkerchief to help filter out the dust until the dust storm passes.

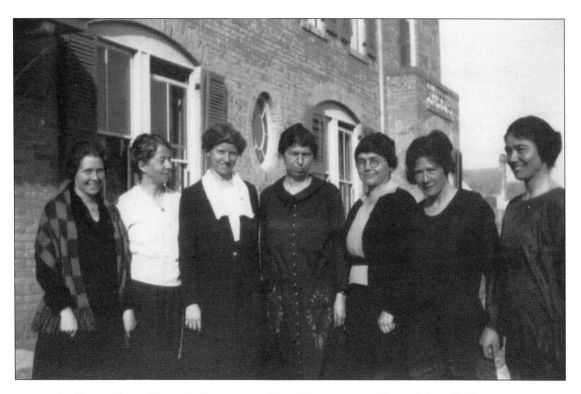

Ladies at Grace House in Dec. 1923: Myra Sawyer, nurse (second from left), Alice Reed, principal of Girls School (center), Mabel Huggins, teacher, Anne Pendleton, visiting sister-in-law, and Lois (right end).

In April 1919 Alice Reed served as a delegate to the annual meeting of the Shantung mission held in Lintsing. She travelled by Peking cart (a two wheeled cart without springs or seats, pulled by a donkey or mule) the 60 miles, a two or three day journey along rutted dirt roads. After spending the night camping in a rural inn where travelers and animals sleep together, they rose at dawn and found a rather strong south wind blowing. It was refreshing at first, but before long a real dust storm was blowing, one that lasted two days. "After the noon-day rest we passed through a sandy area where the sand blew so that we sat inside the cart, held down the front curtain, and covered our eyes and nose with our handkerchiefs. The air was so full of dust we couldn't see the ground ten feet away and the carter lost the road! We reached Lintsing at five o'clock and were glad to be there, I assure you. We did some thorough washing including washing our hair. Then I put on cold cream on my face which was fairly sand-papered in spots."

Dust storms also occur in October and November and through the dry winter months. In early November 1920, Alice Reed wrote: "There were terrific dust storms Tuesday and Wednesday and wind coming from the south. Then in the afternoon there was a lull for half an hour when it was oppressively warm.

Then a cloud of dust came from the north with a worse wind than that from the south had been. It was the worst wind I have seen in China."

In March of 1922 a terrific dust storm followed eight days of strong winds. The dust storms usually decrease in frequency in May when the spring and summer rains begin, enabling a good winter wheat crop and prospects for good summer crops. However on May 18, 1924, Alice Reed wrote: "This has developed into a grey, dusty day which would be very hot except that the dust hides the sun. The thermometer outside registers just 90 and the thermometer indoors not quite 80. It reached 105 before the day was over."

Influenza Epidemic of 1918

Alice Reed wrote from Tehchow on October 18, 1918: "Every day all last week 3 or 4 girls were taken sick with a cough, sore throat and high fever. We heard that the same thing was going through the city and every house on the long South Suburb street had someone sick. Many shops were unable to do business. On Sunday when Dr. Metcalf went to the hospital she found that the hospital accountant had died. She said he wasn't sick enough to die. So she wired Mr. Green at the Rockefeller Foundation (Peking Union Medical College) in Peking to send medical help. She was the only foreign medical doctor at Tehchow at the time. She spent the morning on throat cultures and thought one looked like plague. That is what worried her so. She immediately ordered all who were well to wear masks. We American women worked all day making masks, each putting on the first she made. But it was too late to do me any good for I already had a fever and was put to bed before supper. Dr. Miles arrived that evening and a doctor from Peking the next day. They calmed our fears as to the danger of plague and said it was influenza (flu). Some of the people at the hospital had fever up to 106 degrees. The highest I got was 103.2 degrees. The three Chinese doctors and all but two of the fifteen or more nurses had it. School was closed for a week. Business in the city has been paralyzed and shop keepers have been terrified lest while they were sick robbers should come to Tehchow. Government schools are closed. We had no church services. It is as if a week had dropped out of the year. I taught an English class this morning. The girls still look pale and from the way they cough I think I won't try to start a music class for a while."

November 3, 1918: "There has been a two year old at the hospital lately with the following: influenza, pneumonia, whooping cough, malaria, dysentery, and worms. Needless to say he nearly died but is getting well now."

January 19, 1919: "The influenza has been much worse in America than it was here and you have had the anxiety of it so long. Of course no one will ever

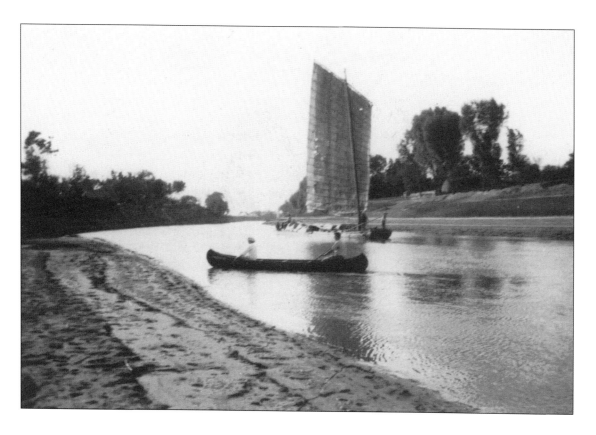

Lois and John Decker (teacher from Grinnell) paddling her canoe "Wawataysee" on the Grand Canal, Tehchow. Native sailboat in distance.

know how many Chinese had it or died of it, but at least it was not so serious among foreigners out here as it was in America."

Drought

TEHCHOW, May 23, 1920: "Drought continues. The winter wheat between us and the city continues to ripen. Apparently only the land which was flooded two years ago has any wheat on it."

TEHCHOW, May 30, 1920: "The wheat between us and the city was being harvested this morning and it was an interesting sight. It was not cut, but pulled up by the roots and tied into bundles all by hand. No sooner had one field been harvested, than gleaners who had been waiting at the edge of the field swarmed over it like a flock of huge blue crows, and they each seemed to find a little bunch of wheat. I heard today that the drought extends into Shansi on the west and Manchuria and Mongolia on the north."

TEHCHOW, August 22, 1920: "There has been only a little rain all summer so the crops are almost a complete failure. It is a distressing sight with corn only about six inches high or tasseling at a foot and a half, millet three inches high, and in some places the ground is bare, showing that the seed never sprouted. Millet is four or five times as expensive as a year ago, wheat more than twice. Already a family to the south of us has taken poison to escape starvation. There is food to be had, but people have no money with which to buy it."

"Grain is being brought in by train from south of the Yellow River. The governor of our province has sent some money to this area. In some places whole families have gathered up their few possessions and started off. I saw one such family last Wednesday. The father was pushing a wheelbarrow on which there were a few small bundles and two little children. Behind came the mother and a little boy, seven perhaps, who was entirely guiltless of clothing."

TEHCHOW, September 5, 1920: "The famine area extends to the north and west. Investigators say that several hundred thousand will starve to death in our Tehchow field unless they are given help. We are appealing to both the Chinese and the American Red Cross, though we must try not to let the sad state of affairs get on our nerves for we will need all our energy before the year is over."

TEHCHOW, October 10, 1920: "Eight thousand dollars has just been sent for famine relief. This will be used as loans for people to buy seed wheat. If people are too poor to plant wheat now they will still have to be fed through next summer."

TEHCHOW, November 15, 1920: "Plans for relief go slowly. The Red Cross has authorized spending five thousand dollars for road repair which will give temporary employment to sixty men. Thirty small boys of destitute families in one of the worst areas have been brought to our Boys' School where they will be housed, fed, taught part of the day and given some industrial work. We hope to do the same thing at our Girls' School."

TEHCHOW, December 5, 1920: "Paul MacEachron of our mission has charge of the commissary for all the Red Cross work in this region where half a million dollars is being put into road building. Helen is teaching his classes and Mr. Wang largely manages the school. Recruiting the workmen is the hardest job in some ways. There has to be careful investigation to be sure only the neediest are taken."

TEHCHOW, January 23, 1921: "Chinese business men have a soup kitchen in the city where they feed about four thousand daily, giving each a portion of millet porridge each morning. The American Red Cross is now feeding forty-five thousand people. We'll be feeding one hundred and fifty thousand people before a month has passed. Our mission is giving help in the area east of the railway, which the Red Cross doesn't touch."

Pneumonic Plague Epidemic of 1921

TEHCHOW, March 10, 1921: "Last Friday pneumonic plague was discovered at Sang Yuan fifteen miles north of here. Since then there has been a more or less continuous stream of doctors and telegrams. The doctors going into the area needed plague suits, so several of us spent Sunday making them. It was decided that no one should go to church in the city. In fact our compound is in partial quarantine. There have been about ninety deaths to date, but as the weather is getting warm it won't continue long."

TEHCHOW, March 27, 1921: "Dr. Yu of the Board of Interior, a very fine man, died of plague this week. He confessed that he had pushed down his mask when looking at a boy who had recently died, thinking the boy had been dead really longer than he had. Nine men, mostly doctors, all Chinese except one Frenchman, who had been living with Dr. Yu have been in quarantine until today when the period of incubation ended. And they are all right, so we are all glad. It was a marvel they escaped."

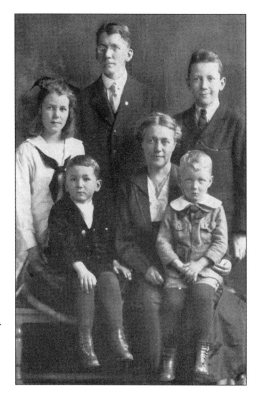

Tucker family in Tehchow, 1919: Dr. Francis Tucker (hospital superintendent), his wife Dr. Emma Tucker and their four children, all of whom became physicians.

During the epidemic of pneumonic plague in Tehchow in March 1921, the missionaries made soup to feed the plague victims. A picture of the missionaries making the plague soup shows Dr. Lois Pendleton and Alice Reed and others on the staff making the soup and feeding the plague victims.

FAMINE RELIEF COMMISSION

"There has been a great drive through China to raise funds for famine relief. A million and a half Chinese dollars has been secured so far, which is good for poor old China. With all the generous help and relief that have come in, conditions are better than we had hoped they would be. Perhaps we underestimated the ability of the Chinese to live on make-shifts and hope. At any rate there have been no wholesale deaths from starvation, only those who are weak and sick, and babies. The misery is great but the Chinese are used to being miserable."

Dr. Francis Tucker of the Tehchow mission served as head of the Famine Relief Commission of Shantung Province. Oliver Julian Todd was one of the

American engineers who went to China in 1920 to work for the Red Cross and the Famine Relief Commission to build roads and dikes; to rebuild the Grand Canal; to "harness" the Yellow River and thus prevent the major floods which destroyed hundreds of thousands of square miles of farms; and to provide famine relief. Major O.J. (Oliver Julian) Todd met regularly with Dr. Tucker regarding the projects and stayed as a guest at Grace House in the mission compound at Tehchow.

PEI TAI HO

Americans working in north China spent their summer holiday at Pei Tai Ho (Beidaihe), the summer beach resort east of Peking on the coast of the Yellow Sea. It was a ten hour, all day train ride 150 to 200 miles from Peking via Tientsin, with a delightful sea-breeze after leaving Tientsin. There were about three hundred summer cottages and private homes in Pei Tai Ho, scattered in three areas: Rocky Point, East Cliff, and West End.

Alice Reed described Pei Tai Ho in a letter to her family: "The shore is irregular with a succession of small bays which are separated by rocky promontories where waves continually break over the rocks. In the bays are beautiful sandy beaches. The hill that rises gradually for about half a mile is covered with little gray brick cottages as wood is too expensive to use. A few of the larger houses have wood verandas around them. The people in our neighborhood are nearly all missionaries, but there are business and diplomatic people also, some of whom come from as far away as Shanghai. There is a hall (community center) in the middle of Pei Tai Ho that is used for church services on Sunday and for various kinds of meetings during the week."

There were no paved roads or motor vehicles, only donkey paths and trails, with donkeys providing transportation in this quiet fishing village and peaceful resort.

"We went swimming in the little bay just a few minutes walk from our cottage. The water is cold in June but fine and invigorating. In the afternoon we walked to East Cliff, about two miles, and stayed to a picnic supper where we met some fine people—mostly women, however, as the men bring their wives and children, then most of them go back for a month or more of work in Peking. We rode home on donkeys, which do a flourishing business."

ShanHaiKuan, a port about ten miles northeast of Pei Tai Ho, is a place where the mountains come close to the sea. The Great Wall follows along these mountains at the northern border of China and then crosses the plain a few miles to end at the sea. It is a short train ride from Pei Tai Ho to ShanHaiKuan. Here tourists take donkeys for the ride up the mountain to a small temple surrounded by pine trees with a fine view across the plain to the sea.

Another favorite outing from Pei Tai Ho was a trip to the sand dunes. Alice Reed's description: "The weather being fine, a group of us took some fruit, sandwiches, hard-boiled eggs and coffee, and riding donkeys went to the sand dunes which are about three or four miles beyond East Cliff (northeast) and which are as interesting as anything I have ever seen. Recent rain made the dunes easy to walk over and climb."

Two of the favorite picnic spots within Pei Tai Ho were Lighthouse Point and Lotus Hill. Julian wrote in his diary, "Wednesday evening we had a picnic at Lighthouse Point. We walked home the two and a half miles along the beach and then had a swim. The moon had gone down, but the phosphorescence in the water was wonderful. I think magnificent would not be too strong a word. Sparks like fire scattered from our hands as we passed them through the water. And as we walked, it was almost as if our feet had electric lights on them."

POLITICAL TURMOIL

In September 1918 robbers and bandits presented a major problem in Shantung province. Alice Reed wrote, "Robbers have been much worse this last month than at any time before, and in a good many places people don't dare stay in their houses at night but take their children and hide in the cornfields. Travel is so unsafe that it is impossible to hire a cart. I was afraid our girl stu-

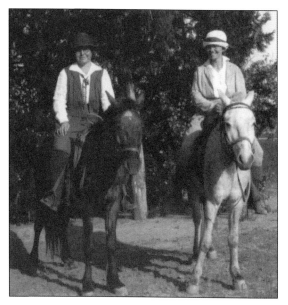

Lois and Mabel riding their horses, Tehchow, May 1923.
Below: Lois and Mabel Huggins in Tehchow, May 1923.

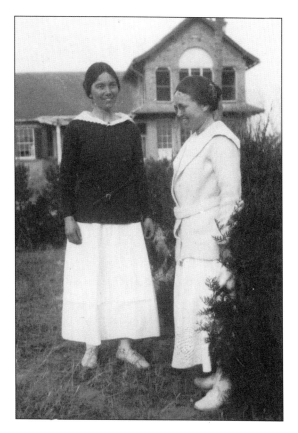

dents would be unable to come, but the parents are glad to get them here to a safe place. One girl walked forty miles dressed as a boy, accompanied by a woman dressed as a beggar and a man who came as a peanut vendor. Officials have given people permission to protect themselves with firearms. We are trying to impress the Chinese government and the American legation that something must be done. Banditry was usually worse when the crops were tall and until they were cut."

In August 1919 political conditions in Shantung had reached a bad state, as pro-Japanese militarists had gotten control and gave harsh treatment to students and other patriotic Chinese who boycotted Japanese goods. The Japanese also tried to stir up feeling against Americans.

In April 1922 clashes occurred between the soldiers of rival warlords, Chang TsoLin and Wu BeiFu. Preparations for fighting included tearing up the railroad track to the north of Tehchow for a mile or so, so there were no regular through trains.

Quotations from Alice Reed's letters, which follow, present a detailed picture of turmoil and suffering in China in the 1920's:

TEHCHOW, October 12, 1924: "Some people stayed at Pei Tai Ho until fighting had begun at ShanHaiKuan to the northeast. They could look across the bay and see airplanes dropping bombs. These last people were taken away by steamer as train service had stopped. Yesterday's paper reports that three days of heavy fighting, with much suffering, and probably a victory for Chang TsoLin, the Manchurian warlord. Friday was the anniversary of the establishment of the Republic, but the distressing conditions in the country meant little enthusiasm for celebrating. The schools had a holiday with a patriotic program, but the speakers were rather at a loss to find something to say. However other republics have had a slow, hard beginning. Not a great deal of progress can be expected in thirteen years."

"The three marauders of last spring appealed to Tsinan and have been released, so our teachers are very uneasy and not at all sure they are willing to stay on. We have a watchman all the time and a dog with two puppies which are something of a comfort to the teachers."

TEHCHOW, October 25, 1924: "All week men have been impressed into military service, not as soldiers but as laborers to dig trenches at the front. Soldiers go to the villages and take any able-bodied man they see until they have secured the quota for that village. It is terrifying to the people as they have no interest in helping their country and there is no financial recompense. Mr. Matthews was horseback riding the other day and as he went through villages he heard doors and gates slamming shut. People supposed he was a soldier coming to seize them."

"Feng YuHsiang (the Christian General) is reported to have sealed up Peking, supposedly as an act of disloyalty to the central government which he was supposed to be supporting. If it is true, I'm afraid there will be fighting in Peking."

TEHCHOW, November 2, 1924: "The Chinese, and we foreigners too, have been quite excited over Feng YuHsiang's defection or coup. He had the support of a good many provinces and planned to make terms with Chang TsoLin after the rendering of Wu BeiFu helpless and so end the civil war. Wu was not as weak as Feng thought, although he had been defeated by Chang. And it looks as if he will be able to fight Feng."

TEHCHOW, November 14, 1924: "Railroad connections both to the north and the south of us have been broken for two weeks, but mail began coming in by Tsingtao two days ago. We are peaceful here although it looked for awhile as if there might be fighting in this area. Tehchow is a strategic city because of the arsenal located there."

"The Chinese have been greatly distressed about the impressing of carts and men. Some of the horrors of war were related to us by one of these men who is back from the front at ShanHaiKuan. His duty was to carry food up to the trenches and bring back the wounded. He said more were dying of hunger than in battle. And those who were considered hopeless were shot by their own men. He deserted, making his escape along with others part of whom were regular soldiers."

TEHCHOW, June 7, 1925: "The Daily is full of trouble in Shanghai. It apparently started with a strike in Japanese cotton mills. A Chinese laborer was killed and students took up the matter, holding mass meetings in the street. Feeling ran so high that the police, under the British Municipal Council, felt it necessary to disperse the mob and in doing so seven students were killed. There has been a lot of rioting since then. Students all over China are stopping their classes and devoting their time to mass meetings and various kinds of publicity. The students are demanding return of all the foreign concessions, the abolition of extraterritoriality, and punishment of the police that killed the students. No one knows what the outcome will be, but it is certainly a most deplorable affair."

TEHCHOW, June 14, 1925: "Student demonstrations have spread like wildfire. And practically all the high schools and colleges in the country have struck, giving their time to speaking, distributing literature and the like. Word reached our schools yesterday. The China Daily was suppressed two weeks ago for pro Wu BeiFu remarks, which delayed the information getting to our students. It was only when a letter came from Peking addressed to the student body that they got excited. At first the girls thought they wanted to stop all school work. Then they decided they would like to take their final examinations, but carry on propaganda on the side."

"The Chinese teachers take charge of the student activities. Although the movement is anti-British only, national feeling is running high, and it is well for an American to keep in the background. We Americans are glad that America holds no concessions, but we do have extra-territorial privileges along with other foreigners. I am sure that the girls are just as friendly toward me as ever, but with the feeling running so high I am very careful as to what I say and am letting the Chinese teachers take the lead."

TEHCHOW, June 28, 1925: "A recent letter from Shanghai reports that soldiers and police are very conspicuous, and few shops are open. A great effort is being made to force the British and the Japanese to give up their concessions through boycotting their businesses as well as British mission schools. The Japanese hospital in Tsinan is closed. It is remarkable how much the students have been able to accomplish. And if China had any kind of a decent government, it would be an easy matter for her to recover her conceded lands and get new treaties with foreign countries."

TEHCHOW, October 18, 1925: "The papers say there is danger of war breaking out around Shanghai. We are hoping it may be averted, but railroad connections between Shanghai and Nanking have already been broken."

TEHCHOW, December 11, 1925: "This is the fifth day of battle that has been raging west of the city, just two miles from our compound here. We have been in no immediate danger and only one bullet is known to have dropped in the compound. Still it has been a tense week, and it is a relief to have the firing growing gradually less today. This is part of the struggle for supremacy that has been going on between the generals, or warlords, for the last two months. About three weeks ago a conference was held at which the three important generals (Wu Bei Fu, Chang Tso Lin and Feng Yu Hsiang) came to an important agreement on their 'spheres of influence', whereby Shantung was to be ceded from Chang to Wu. Shortly after, we heard that Governor Chang of this province was a friend and relative of General Chang who was refusing to withdraw from Shantung and defeated Wu's troops that came in from Honan. We suppose that it is the other Honan troops that have come to try to get possession of the arsenal west of the city."

"Tuesday evening there was additional excitement due to the fact that bandits were reported near to us on the east. A number of the students in our

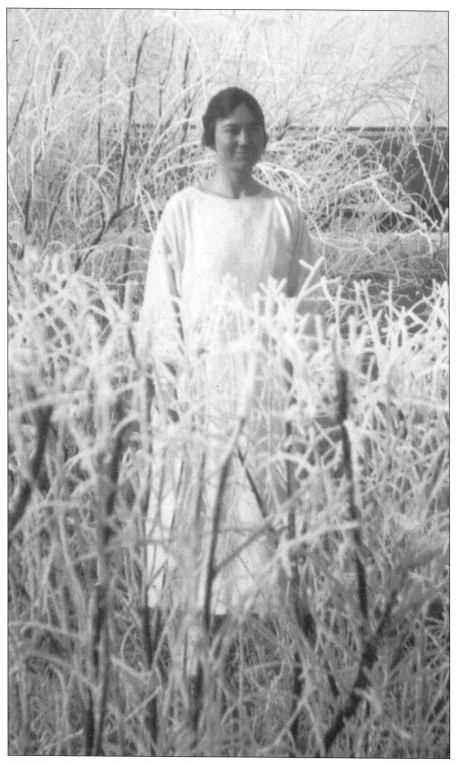

Lois in winter wool uniform in hoarfrost, Tehchow, 1924.

Boys School have had fathers carried off or killed by the bandits. And it is understood that the bandits are wanting to get a hold of one particular boy who reported to the local magistrate the killing of his father and uncles, and after identifying one of the guilty bandits saw him beheaded at the magistrate's order. The boys are greatly alarmed and afraid to go to bed until a sentry of teachers and students was arranged for the night in two hour shifts."

"The Honan troops are reported to have withdrawn to the northwest and we hope they are gone for good, except that the people here hate Governor Chang heartily and would rather be under Wu. Of course this is a republic, but just at present that has little effect upon who has control of what region."

TEHCHOW, December 13, 1925: "More than seven hundred refugees are in the compound, some from fear of fighting, some fleeing the bandits, and some from fear of future looting by soldiers. The Chinese felt that they would be safe in our compound, as was quite certainly true, but we insisted that the people bring only necessary clothing, bedding and food, but no valuables. Honan troops trying to surround the city by circling to the north and east were met by Chang's troops to the north of our compound where a skirmish took place. Bullets flew through the compound but no one was hit."

"This morning we got news of the night's events. Chang's troops fled during the night, doing some looting as they left, and leaving the city to the Honan troops. Dr. Tucker went into the city with a nurse and first aid supplies. He found a lot of wounded soldiers to bring out to our hospital. Two of our American men went to nearby villages in search of wounded and brought a few to the hospital."

TEHCHOW, December 15, 1925: "Can you imagine what it would be like to try to run a boarding school (and a hospital) in the middle of a battle field? That is what we were doing yesterday. Honan troops had occupied all the villages to the south and east of us, in case Chang's troops should return. This very thing happened and the fighting began about eleven in the morning and lasted until dark. It didn't look like the kind of battle I've seen in pictures, but was a series of skirmishes with from ten to fifty soldiers running from one protected spot to another, stopping to fire and then running again. They were on all sides of our compound, but mostly to the south. Many bullets flew through the yard, a window in the Matthews house was struck, and a bullet whizzed by my head as I went back to school in the afternoon. It was a peculiar sound, but I had no difficulty in deciding what it was; it landed on the ground several rods ahead of me."

"The last class before noon was turned into a session for making bandages for the hospital as it was impossible to keep the girls at their lessons. Firing was close and continuous after lunch, so all we tried to do was to keep the girls occupied and out of danger. We played games for a while and finally had classes for an hour. I had my girls sitting on the floor so as to have the protection of the brick walls. It was wearing to say the least. Fighting decreased as dark came on, and we learned that the city had been retaken by Chang's troops. The Honan troops withdrew to the west of the river (Canal) and the city was looted again as it had been by the withdrawal of Chang's troops."

"Chang's troops had gathered up two hundred of the bandits that have been making trouble to the east and used them in yesterday's attack. Their being in the city has caused much alarm among civilians; this was a threat to soldiers at the main gate of our compound to loot the compound, and has provided this day with its special anxiety. Four of our best men, two Chinese and two American, made two trips into the city and finally got assurance of the general that we would be protected. Some girls helped at the hospital as did Mabel and I the latter part of the afternoon."

TEHCHOW, December 19, 1925: "The hospital has one hundred and seven patients, twenty three Chang's soldiers, fifty Honan soldiers, and the rest with a few exceptions are civilians who were accidentally wounded. I have been helping at the hospital every day after school. Help is especially needed at meal times as there are many who can not feed themselves. The cases are nearly all serious, and practically everyone must have an operation sooner or later."

TEHCHOW, March 21, 1926: "The fighting this side of Tientsin is continuing, and a military train goes south each night carrying wounded soldiers to Tsinan or Tsingtao. Chang's warships have reached the river, the Tientsin harbor, so the city is completely isolated."

"The strong patriotic feeling that is running through all schools in China has expressed itself here in faithful devotion to school work and a desire for social service in the community. Beside helping in the church school and in the hospital, the high school girls are continuing the charity school for village children that was started more than two years ago. The industrial department in our school provides work for some of our more needy girls. There are thirty five who could not be here in school were it not for the money they earn doing filet crochet as applied to household linens. There is a ready market for their work among American and British residents in Tientsin and Peking, and among summer resort people at Pei Tai Ho."

TEHCHOW, September 20, 1926: "Fighting is reported to be beginning at An Hui between Wu Bei Fu's men and Chang Tso Lin's. Wu holds the southwest, Feng the northwest, and Chang all the eastern area."

TEHCHOW, November 2, 1926: "Various societies have been organized through the country for protection from bandits. To the east of us there is a rather strong one called the Red Gun Society. These are something like the old Boxer societies whose members claim to be immune to bullets. They are not contrary to law in themselves, but usually do not get on well with the military, as they accuse the latter of being 'in' with the bandits. The ninth of September, the local military started east avowedly to attack the bandits, gathering supplies forcibly from villages as they went along. When people in one village objected, they shot several of the villagers. It so stirred the people that they gathered the Red Gun Society members of the region and attacked and defeated the soldiers."

"Since then there have been threats from both sides, and attempts to settle the matter too, and we thought the affair was quieting down. But a week ago soldiers went east where they attacked, defeated, and burned the villages. We had seen the troops going east and the next day heard firing all day: rifles, machine guns, and small cannons. That night we sent word to our local official to ask permission to go out and get the wounded, but he said we would have to wait until the affair was over. The next day we could see the smoke of burning villages all day. Of course the walls are adobe but the roofs burn and all fuel the villages had stored and the grain on the threshing floor and the like were burned. We began to see soldiers returning with loot, and that has gone on ever since. Saturday permission was given for our people from our mission compound to go out to investigate the condition, on the condition that only Chinese go. The latter say the officials are ashamed to let us see what has been done. Plans were made and ten groups of investigators went out on Sunday. They found the villages, about a dozen near here and many more farther east, absolutely deserted. Not a chicken or a dog made a noise as they passed through. We suppose that all the living had fled to other villages. All animals had been taken by the soldiers. They found dead villagers, one hundred in one village and nearly as many in the others. The dead included women and children. Only five wounded were found and brought to our hospital. I suppose thousands have fled from their homes and will return to find their homes burned and their winter supply of grain and fuel gone, in fact everything gone. It is almost impossible to realize the suffering it has caused. In a way this is the worst thing that has struck Tehchow yet."

LINTSING, March 27, 1927: "The Daily yesterday reported the fall of Shanghai to the Nationalist forces under Chiang Kai Shek and that southern Nationalist troops are pressing on to Nanking. The news is not very recent as it is slow getting into Lintsing. We wondered what the later developments were; we wondered still more when at 7:30 in the evening a telegram came from our American consul in Tsinan instructing American women and children to withdraw to Tientsin immediately. A reply has been sent asking for more information. We are pushing through Association business so we can get back to Techow on Tuesday. If anything is going to happen, Alfred Heininger and I, principals of the two boarding schools, should be there to make plans for the schools. We have had it in mind for some time that work might have to be handed over to the Chinese at almost any time. And things are in pretty good shape to do this."

TEHCHOW, April 3, 1927: "The future is very uncertain, and it is hard to know what we should do. Mothers and children have all gone, or will go as soon as they can. The Chinese Christians here do not anticipate any trouble, and I think it would look to them like running off if we should all withdraw. On the other hand Christians in Peking and Tientsin are telling missionaries that they are going to be more of a liability than an asset until this revolution is over and that they had better withdraw."

We feel fairly certain that southern troops will loot all foreign houses, so we are having to consider what to take and what to leave. I haven't started packing as I am hoping later news will give us a more intelligent basis for action, that is whether it seems we will be away a few months or a few years. However I am sorting things and burning old letters. It is a strange state of affairs. On the one hand we are planning how to pack, and on the other hand we go right on planning for next fall term and buying new textbooks."

TIENTSIN, April 17, 1927: "People of all missions and nationalities, and business people in interior places, have all withdrawn to port cities. We had informal mission meetings the first of the week and agreed that people who do not go home, those who's furloughs are due this year or next, should go to Korea rather than stay in port cities. We don't want to put ourselves under the protection of American gunboats and soldiers. There are one hundred seventy five foreign battleships in Chinese waters now and thousands of troops, all of which does not make for harmonious international relations."

"The southern Nationalist troops have met with reversals recently so will not be coming on north as rapidly as some feared. A number of men are going back to their stations to carry on their work or get things in better shape. If the Chinese can get things in good shape before trouble comes it may save mission work from being completely upset. Our problem now will be to keep funds from America coming until the transition period is past."

FURLOUGH YEAR (1925-1926)

Dr. Lois Pendleton had furlough in America from June 1925 to June 1926. During this time she met at the American Board (A.B.C.F.M.) office in

Boston to report on her work at Tehchow; she traveled to various Congregational Churches around the U.S. to tell about her work at the mission station in Tehchow; and visited her mother and sister in Claremont following the death of her father.

When Lois returned to China, her mother and Adaline, now nine, went with her. While crossing the Pacific by steamship, they stopped in Hawaii to visit missionary friends. In Japan they visited more friends at Kobe College, and went sightseeing in scenic Kyoto and Nara.

Upon arrival in Tientsin they traveled directly to Tehchow. When Lois was able to get some time off from the hospital, she took Mother (in sedan chair) and Adaline to climb the sacred mountain, Tai Shan, and to Chu-fu, birth place of Confucius. She also introduced them to Peking, visiting historic places as well as Peking Union Medical College (Rockefeller Foundation). Lois took time for a meeting with Dr. Wood, a neurologist at P.U.M.C., to consult with him regarding cases of toxoplasmosis she had seen and cared for at the hospital in Tehchow.

Mother Pendleton and Adaline remained at Tehchow with Lois about six months, until after Thanksgiving 1926. Then they went by ship to the Philippines to visit Robert and Anne at their home at Los Baños College of Agriculture, where they stayed for the next fifteen months.

MEDICAL CHALLENGES

The medical challenges at the mission station in Tehchow were tremendous and varied, because patients came to the hospital as a last resort. When all else failed, including the local herbalist, and the family was sure the patient was about to die, they came. The critically ill or injured and dying were brought from miles around on wooden carts or wheelbarrows over rutted dirt roads. In addition to infants and children starving during times of famine, there were babies and children suffering malnutrition because of heavy infestations of intestinal parasites. Some of these patients could be treated medically with anti- parasitic chemicals. Others required surgery because the parasites caused intestinal obstruction.

Epidemic diseases in addition to intestinal parasites included malaria, typhoid, rabies, tetanus (very common cause of death in newborns because the umbilical cord in home deliveries was cut with scissors which had not been sterilized), pneumonic plague and tuberculosis. Miliary tuberculosis, cavitary pulmonary tuberculosis, and tuberculosis of the bone were all very common in children as well as adults. The lack of x-ray equipment to aid with diagnosis was a distinct disadvantage.

Orthopedic injuries such as fractures were commonly neither set nor cast, resulting often in severe orthopedic deformities. So many people with crippling deformities would come to the mission hospital in hopes of having their old deformities corrected.

During her years as physician and surgeon at the Tehchow mission hospital, one of Dr. Lois' most difficult challenges occurred one day when a farmer brought his horse to the hospital for treatment. He was politely told that the hospital provided medical care for people, not for animals. The farmer was undaunted and insisted that his horse be treated. After all, his horse was his beast of burden, far more valuable to him than any member of his family, including his wife. Dr. Lois was called to the hospital front steps to assess the situation and to deal with the problem. After examining the horse she made the diagnosis of peri-rectal abscess. The horse was obviously in great pain and something needed to be done for him. Being a horse owner herself, she realized that if she did not try, the horse probably would get no help. Furthermore she realized that if she could cure this farmer's horse, the news would get around the region that the new American physician was skilled and could cure her patients. Perhaps patients would be less apprehensive about coming to the mission hospital.

Although she knew little about the anatomy of the horse (having studied no veterinary medicine), she decided to treat the horse as if it were a human and proceeded with the surgery. She sent for the nurse anesthetist to administer drop ether by gauze sponge to the horse's nostrils, after getting several strong men with heavy ropes to hold the horse down on the ground. Then Dr. Lois proceeded to surgically remove the peri-rectal abscess. Fortunately the horse recovered nicely, the farmer was very grateful, and her reputation as a skillful surgeon spread throughout the region.

An astonishing surgical case she had at Tehchow was a lady who was brought many miles by wheelbarrow with her airway nearly obstructed by a huge mass on her neck. A goiter in her thyroid gland had grown so large that, when it was surgically removed, it filled a wash basin. This case was documented in the photograph album Dr. Lois Pendleton kept of her most interesting surgical cases.

Since patients came for help only when they were in a very serious condition, the work was more demanding than the same patient load at a dispensary-hospital in America. Nearly all the patients required surgery. They included tumors, cancers, goiters, tubercular bones, broken bones that had grown together crooked, abscesses, skull fractures, gunshot wounds and severe burns. With the civil wars, guerrilla skirmishes, and bandit raids there were many war casualties, both soldiers and civilians, who needed medical care. Hospital equipment was

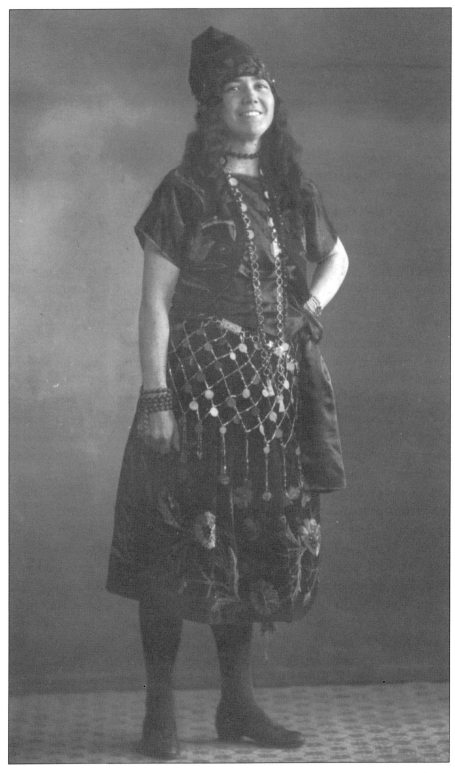

"Once she was a Gypsy maiden" . . . *February, 1924 costume party at Tehchow when she met O. J. Todd, civil engineer.*

very meager and limited. Like x-ray equipment, anesthesia machines had not yet become available. I.V. solutions, blood and plasma were not available in prepared bottles. So when such things were needed the medical staff simply improvised with ingredients available from the kitchen and from live donors.

When the second son of Harold and Grace Matthews was born at the Tehchow hospital, Dr. Lois delivered the baby and immediately recognized that the baby was suffering from Rh incompatibility. She did an exchange transfusion directly to the infant from his father, Harold Matthews. The baby thrived and the Matthews were very grateful. This was the first known exchange transfusion attempted in a mission hospital in China. The baby, Burtus Matthews, grew up to become a physician.

CELEBRATION OF HOLIDAYS
July 4th

American missionaries in north China usually celebrated July 4th at Pei Tai Ho with baseball games in the afternoon, picnic supper on the shore, and a band concert and fireworks after dark. They sang "Star Spangled Banner," "America," "Columbia, the Gem of the Ocean," and "Over There" and felt quite patriotic. An American military band stationed at ChingWanTao, about twelve miles northeast of Pei Tai Ho, came to play in the Assembly Hall. The concert was followed by a spectacular fireworks display at the seashore after sunset.

Costume Party

In February, 1924 a successful costume party was held in the mission compound. All of the Americans working in the Tehchow region were invited, including the engineers working for the Famine Relief Commission. Among these was Oliver Julian Todd. Dr. Lois, dressed as a gypsy, caught his eye. Courtship developed following this party, eventually leading to their marriage in 1927 in the Philippines.

Thanksgiving

The missionaries always celebrated Thanksgiving although their mission schools did not have a holiday. By adjusting their teachers' schedules, everyone had the middle of the day free. They had a Thanksgiving Service at Grace House (where Dr. Lois and Alice Reed lived) at 12:30 followed by Thanksgiving Dinner at 1:30 PM at the MacEachron's house or at the Heininger's house. Eighteen were gathered at the table to enjoy roast bustard (instead of turkey, as turkeys were not readily available). A bustard is a big wild bird with a long neck, much larger than a goose. They served it with noodles or rice, sweet potatoes, and green vegetables. A favorite dessert was "Peking Dust", made of ground roasted chestnuts folded into whipped cream.

Christmas

The cold winter weather arrived in Tehchow and the furnaces were turned on for the first time sometime between Thanksgiving and Christmas. The winter of 1919 the furnace boiler cracked and was creatively repaired by Mr. Wolf (the architect and builder for all the A.B.C.F.M. mission stations) with oatmeal gruel. The thin oatmeal gruel he put in the boiler stopped the leak and the missionaries were able to have heat the winter of 1919-1920. Ah, Yankee ingenuity.

In December 1923 turkeys were running around the mission compound being fattened for Christmas dinner. A Chinese farmer who lived between Tehchow and Tientsin began raising turkeys for Americans. Missionaries at Tehchow were able to buy some turkeys several weeks before Christmas, bring them to Tehchow on the train, and fatten them on corn for a few weeks, before butchering them for Christmas dinner.

Packages arrived from home usually in time for Christmas, adding to the festivities. There were special Christmas programs at church and at schools. Christmas services were held at 11:00 AM at the church in South Suburb both on December 24th and 25th. The school girls sang the processional, "O, Come All Ye Faithful", singing a capella in three parts. Christmas breakfast was at Grace House with a tree for the mission children. But instead of giving gifts to each other, the missionaries took money offerings to the church for the poor.

TEHCHOW, December 28, 1924: Alice Reed wrote: "Christmas is past and it was a busy, happy time. There has never been a year when gifts from home arrived in such good time. I saved mine and opened them Christmas eve after I got back from the program at school. The tree here was ready with its decorations and gifts for Christmas morning. The poinsettia, which I have nursed since last year, opened just in time to add to our decorations."

LETTER FROM LOIS PENDLETON, M.D., June 6, 1922

"Dear Friends:

The innumerable demands upon one's time aside from that required for language study and the usual hospital duties preclude the writing of many personal letters to you dear people at the 'home base'.

Summer has come at last. I say 'at last' because my colleagues tell me that this has been a very unusual spring. Thus far it has not been over 100 degrees F in the shade, but it is easily 20 degrees higher in the sun.

The personnel of the Compound is beginning to scatter for the summer. The Tucker family hopes to leave tomorrow for Tungchow to attend the graduation exercises of the Academy, their son William being one of the graduates.

From there the united family will proceed to Pei Tai Ho for the summer (unless Chang TsuLin interferes). Mrs. Bradfield and Master Bobbie have already gone to Tsinan, where Mr. Bradfield will join them for the better half of the summer.

The addition to the hospital, which we call the 'P.W.& S. Building' (private ward and service building), is nearly completed. The name is not quite all-inclusive, for in the second story is the suite for our foreign nurses, Misses Sawyer and Jeune. We are all more thankful than words can express that Miss Jeune has been appointed. We only wish she could be here now to help share the responsibility which is too much for any human being to carry alone, yet what Miss Myra Sawyer (head nurse) has had to shoulder alone for some time.

Nobody that has superintended building operations in the U.S.A. has any idea of the close supervision that is necessary in connection with the building of foreign buildings in China. If Dr. Francis Tucker's letters have been less frequent than usual this spring let me tell you 'There's a reason.' Not only one reason but many. With the usual administrative work of the hospital, plus considerable medical and surgical work per se, plus the many hours spent on committee work in connection with the Refugee Society which came into being on the eve of the late military disturbance hereabout, plus the added duties with the North China Council of our Mission and as chairman of the Committee for the Forty Year Celebration of the founding of the Mission in Shantung, which was recently held here, any ordinary man would have been completely submerged by the flood—but not Dr. Tucker.

May I take you with me on hospital rounds this a.m.? We won't stop to talk about every patient. But you'll want to know something about a few of them. In the first bed is a toothless, wrinkled-faced old woman of sixty-six who came hobbling in on her bound feet from her home some sixty 'li' (a li equals one third mile) distant. A terrible infection of her hand brought her in. And of course she did not come until she could not stand it any longer. The infection evidently had started as a paronychia of the thumb, but the palmar fascia was involved. It had been neglected for several weeks, and finding that she was also diabetic, it was not surprising that gangrene had set in. The hand had assumed enormous proportions, but we can't tell how much of the thumb can be saved. In spite of her serious condition, her son has been here insisting upon taking his mother home to tend the children and watch the house while the rest of the family go out to harvest the wheat crop. This time we succeeded in keeping her a few days longer, but we often are not so successful. They think as soon as they are a little better that they are ready to go home.

In the next bed by the window where she gets lots of sun light is a young woman with tuberculous hip of advanced stage. She is incurable physically, but oh, so very much more comfortable and happy than when she came. Under the tutelage of our faithful Bible woman she has learned to read the phonetic script, and she has learned something of the Heavenly Father who cares.

Little Chang Lan, a young man of seven years, is in the bed with the Balkan frame on it. The bed with the necessary Thomas splint, pulleys and ropes for swinging it is always a trial to the nurses, for it is prone to look untidy. He is a patient little lad, never complaining except when his dressing is being done, and then he has sufficient cause, I can assure you. On entrance he had four inches of dead, honeycombed tibia projecting from his leg. Such cases of neglect as this, thank God, you never see at home. But here it is not a rare occurrence to see such a thing. The dead bone was full of squirming maggots. And on operation we found these ugly creatures in the bone marrow all the way from the knee to the ankle. It certainly was a disgusting sight. We are hoping that by keeping the leg in Buck's extension so that the bone fragments are in proper alignment, nature may be able to regenerate sufficient bone callous from the periosteum to give him a functioning leg.

Hsiu Jung (Beautiful or Excellent Glory), our Dr. Hsiu's little four year old daughter, is Chang Lan's next door neighbor. You should hear the two of them sing the sweet little hymn Mrs. Wang has taught them. The lively, noisy 'Excellent Glory' is an entirely different child from the lethargic, anemic child that she was on entry. She is convalescing from the dreaded Kala Azar, caused by a trypanosome. The clinical picture is one of progressive anemia and general wasting associated with the tremendous enlargement of the spleen. Sometimes the spleen fills half of the abdominal cavity. We confirmed our diagnosis by finding the Leishman Donovan bodies in the spleen cells obtained by splenic puncture. I should like to see an American child as patiently endure the necessary three weekly intravenous injections. Not long ago she was found with her head all carefully draped in a towel playing nurse. On return from a few days at Tsinan, she informed me that she had 'longed and longed for me until her stomach ached.' I wish you could see her give the little Caesarian baby her bottle. It makes too dear a picture for me to attempt to describe.

In the next bed is a five year old boy who came in with a bladder stone which we removed by operation five days ago. The stone, comparatively speaking, was small, being about the size and shape of a candied almond, with a rough surface. He is not a handsome lad, but he is most lovable and patient.

The beloved only son of an old man of seventy lies in the next bed. He is a handsome little fellow of three years. His trouble was double, complete inguinal hernia. He has had an uneventful convalescence since his operation ten days ago. He is a relative of Mr. Chen who is in charge of the arsenal here. When Mrs. Chen comes to see the little patient, she comes in a spick and span mule cart escorted by outriders.

The next bed has just been vacated by a little girl who had been having relapsing fever. She is the eight year old daughter of one of our sewing women. It is a tropical disease caused by a spirochete and carried (transmitted from one person to another) by bedbugs or lice. It is a very satisfactory disease to treat, for it readily responds to intravenous injections of salvarsan.

In the next bed there is no one at present, but I wish the woman that left it to go home to help in the wheat harvest could have stayed a few more days until her abdominal incision was entirely closed. By suprapubic cystotomy we recovered a hair ornament about four and a half inches long and a third of an inch wide.

We have only one case of entropion in the Porter Hospital now. Entropion (inversion of the eyelids so that the lashes continually scratch the cornea) is one of the most common sequellae of trachoma. Great relief is afforded by a very simple operation of everting the lid by removing a small part of it.

There are several more patients I would like to tell you about, but I presume this is about all you non-medical people can stand.

Miss Tinling, of the World W. C. T. U., who gave a series of lectures recently to our nurses and students, was a patient in the hospital for a few days. I have never seen a more appreciative patient. And just a few days ago we received a check from her for the support of a bed for sick nurses. It so happens that the first nurse to occupy the bed is Miss Chao, who was Miss Tinling's nurse, and whom Miss Tinling has become very fond of.

We are all rejoicing over the help promised by the China Medical Board of the Rockefeller Foundation promised for the next five years, a conditional gift conditioned on the Board (A.B.C.F.M.) giving an equal amount. For some time it has been the hope of the hospital staff that a branch dispensary might be established in the city of Tehchow. It was hoped that it might be invited and largely supported by the well-to-do of the city. About a week ago, at a meeting of business men of the city, which Dr. Tucker attended, one of the men asked if we would not be willing to establish a dispensary in the city. It was evidently his own idea. As you can't hurry the East, it probably will take months to get the work started. In connection with the dispensary, it is our hope to carry on a public health campaign. And we hope to have a street chapel and a special center in the course of time.

Yours in the Master's Service,
LOIS PENDLETON, M.D.

Williams-Porter Hospitals,
Tehchow, Shantung, China."

CHAPTER 5

Wedding and Kweichow

In March 1927 Shanghai fell to the Nationalist forces under Chiang Kai Shek, and the southern Nationalist troops were pressing on to Nanking with the expectation of moving northward to Peking. The American consul instructed the women and children in the mission stations to withdraw to the port city of Tientsin immediately. American gunboats and troops were brought to Tientsin in April to protect the American citizens during the civil war, or to evacuate them if necessary. In early April the Tehchow missionaries sorted and packed their possesions and secured their homes, not knowing whether they would be away months or years, feeling fairly certain that the southerners, i.e. Nationalist troops, would loot all foreign houses.

Among the hospital patients at the Tehchow mission was the Heininger's oldest child, Jean, who was confined to bed with tuberculosis of the spine. She had to be strapped to a frame for the evacuation by train to Tientsin. The American physicians and nurses turned over the total care of patients and administration of the hospitals to their Chinese colleagues and left for Tientsin in compliance with orders from the American consul.

WEDDING IN THE PHILIPPINES

Dr. Lois decided that since she had to leave Tehchow, the break from her medical responsibilities would allow her time to marry Oliver Julian Todd, the American engineer. So she wrote to her mother, Jessie, who with ten year old Adaline had extended their stay in the Philippines with Lois's older brother Robert. She informed her mother of her engagement and her plans to come to the Philippines to be married. She arranged to have the wedding at the home of her brother, Dr. Robert Pendleton, and his wife Anne, on the College of Agriculture campus, University of the Philippines, in Los Baños on July 2, 1927.

In 1918 Robert and Anne had gone to Allahabad, India where he was Professor of Agriculture at the mission college. After several years in India he became Professor of Agriculture at Los Baños College in the Philippines.

Lois arrived in the Philippines on May 19, 1927, to prepare for her wedding. Her mother wrote about Lois:

"She was tired, for the last days at Tehchow were very hard physically, with the breaking up of their homes; and very hard in every other way, in breaking the ties with their faithful co-workers; and not knowing if they would ever return. She wrote how splendidly the Chinese doctors and nurses rose to the situation after the first great shock of the withdrawal of the Americans passed. And she was told by some who passed through Tehchow after she left how well the medical, educational and evangelistic work was going on."

Lois had written to her friends from Tientsin on April 21, 1927:

"These days I have often thought of Jesus' unfinished work. Yet it was 'expedient' for his disciples that he go away. I feel it is the same here with us at this time. I mean I believe it is expedient for us to leave our Chinese colleagues at this time. Our withdrawal does not mean the end of foreign missions, despite the newspaper headings these days. Many of us will be invited back later on. A big sphere of helpful service awaits those who will respond to the call. No doubt there will never again be so many foreign missionaries in China, but fewer will be needed. And we shall hope that few foreigners will be in executive positions.

"It is to be hoped that our government will soon find a way to regain China's confidence and to abrogate the unequal treaties. And we hope that America will stand firm against intervention. These may be dark days, but 'tis darkest just before dawn, and I feel sure that the dawn of a better day for China is near at hand.

"Don't think for a moment our responsibility is over and that we can cease giving; now is the most important time to show our trust in our Chinese friends, and for a time, at least, more financial help rather than less will be needed."

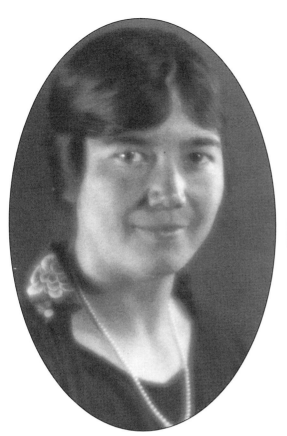 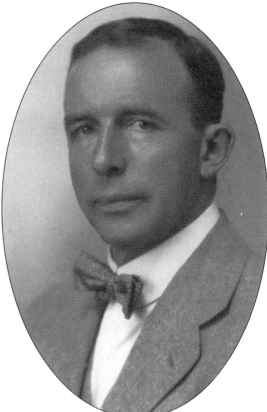

Lois Pendleton age 33 at the time of her marriage in 1927.

Oliver Julian Todd age 47 at the time of his marriage to Lois.

She received many letters from the Chinese doctors in charge at Tehchow, and she was much heartened at the way they were carrying on the work. She was urgently asked to return to Tehchow but declined.

Lois arrived in the Philippines with an engagement ring. Since her work had ended for the present, she felt she could resign from her position at Tehchow. After her marriage she planned to return to China, establishing a home in Peking where her husband, Oliver Julian Todd, civil engineer with the China Famine Relief Commission, would have his head office. She planned to continue her medical work in Peking, doing school health and caring for American missionary patients, as well as doing some clinical teaching at Peking Union Medical College (Rockefeller Foundation), the leading center for western medicine in China.

Before the wedding, time passed quickly with sightseeing trips in the Philippines and weeks of sewing to make lingerie and other items for the bride's

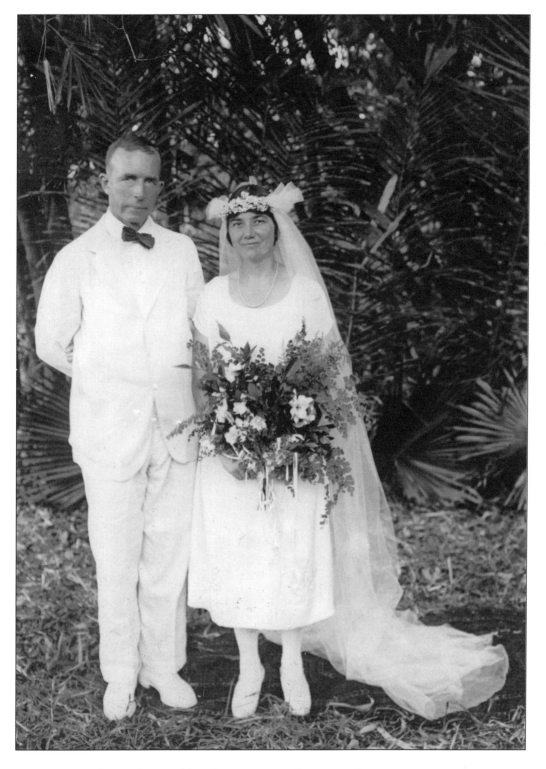

Oliver Julian Todd and Dr. Lois Pendleton on July 2, 1927.

---

trousseau. Anne helped make the trousseau using the beautiful silk and brocade fabrics which Lois had brought from China. All garments including underwear were custom made in the Orient in those days, either sewn by hand or on a sewing machine.

Lois and Julian were married in the bamboo grove in Robert and Anne's garden. It made a beautiful green "wedding bower". The music, including the wedding march, was played on the piano in the house next door. With the windows and louvers open the music wafted across the garden. Professor Roa of the Engineering Department at Los Baños College played the piano beautifully.

Robert and Anne walked with the bride and groom and little Adaline was the ring-bearer for her older sister. Lois's flowers were the lovely gardenias and Maiden Hair fern from Robert and Anne's garden. She wore the veil which Gladys had worn three years earlier when she married Lois's younger brother Morris. Just a few days before the wedding day, the veil arrived by sea mail from Los Angeles. Lois wore a very simple white silk crepe dress, street length and hand embroidered, bought in Shanghai. Although her mother opposed the marriage because Julian was divorced, Jessie wrote: "She was a very handsome bride."

Dr. Rodgers, senior Presbyterian missionary in the Philippines and a warm friend of Robert and Anne, conducted the wedding ceremony about three o'clock in the afternoon. Family and a few close friends were present. At four o'clock a very large reception began in Robert and Anne's home and garden for all the friends and Filipino faculty. There were only twelve Americans present.

About five o'clock, Lois changed into a little brown silk dress with hat and gloves to match and the newlyweds went to Manila. The next morning they took the 8:00 AM train to Baguio, where they enjoyed a honeymoon week. Baguio is a resort in the mountains a day's trip north of Manila at an elevation of 4500 feet among pine trees, where the breeze is cool high above the tropical heat of Manila.

Jessie wrote, "Mr. Todd enjoyed the Baguio country very much, and being a civil engineer, was especially interested in seeing what the American engineers have accomplished there in the mountain roads during the past 25 years. They also made a trip to a paying gold mine, which they were allowed to enter as Mr. Todd was so much interested in the engineering problems."

On Saturday, July 9, Mother Pendleton, Adaline, Robert and Anne went to Manila to have lunch with the bride and groom at the Manila Hotel, and then to the pier to see them off on the *Empress of Asia* for their boat trip to Hongkong and China to embark upon a long and adventuresome wedding trip.

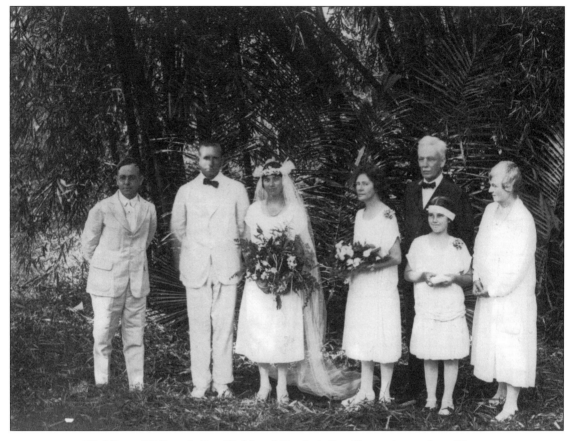

Wedding of Oliver Julian Todd and Dr. Lois Pendleton in garden of her brother Robert's home at Los Baños Agricultural College, Philippines.

WEDDING TRIP TO KWEICHOW

Julian had been invited by the Governor of Kweichow province to come to Kweiyang to build a road for his automobile. Lois and Julian agreed the opportunity to travel to mountainous and remote Kweichow would be a great adventure, even though it would require a month or more of travel on horseback over steep mountain trails, camping wherever they could find shelter. Because of bandits and wet weather it would be a dangerous journey. Both Lois and Julian were fearless, thriving on challenge and adventure, so they decided to go together to Kweichow for an extended journey.

They arrived in Hongkong on July 11, did errands and some sightseeing, then enjoyed two delightful days at Repulse Bay Hotel. Sailing July 16 on "Tonkin" for Haifong, they arrived July 18 and took the afternoon train to Hanoi. After purchasing a saddle the next morning, they went by train to Lokay, continuing to Amichu, and on July 21 traveled on toward Yunnanfu. However broken rail lines and bandit raids caused the train to return to Amichu, where they remained until July 24 when they left for PeiShiChi. They were delayed at TscheTsoun until July 29, then allowed to proceed north on a military train, reaching Yunnanfu that night. On August 2 Julian spent the day on a trip of road inspection to TaPanChiao and back. On August 4 he gave his report and they began packing for their horseback trip to Kweichow. They bought two horses and had them shod, hired five packers, a mafoo (horse attendant or helper) and a travel boy.

The entourage departed early the next morning for Liang. The following day they climbed on foot and by horseback the steep trail, at one point 8,500 feet above sea level, to reach camp at TienShang at 6,300 feet altitude. On August 8 they started out with six new coolies and the same mafoo. The five Yunnanfu coolies had run away at daybreak, considering the journey too rigorous, pace too fast and hours too long. The road was fairly level, mostly 6,200 feet elevation to Makai. The next morning Lois and Julian were up early and waited on a hilltop at 7,400 feet altitude 40 minutes for their military escort of thirty soldiers and coolies to catch up. Nearly every afternoon they were drenched by rain showers and the roads became slippery and wet.

When they left ShihShingHsien they took 100 soldiers with them to protect them from bandits. The trail rose to 6,700 feet before dropping into the LoPing valley where they camped at a temple in ChinLaoHo at an altitude of 5,000 feet. The coolies and horses were tired, so they camped at LoPing. The next morning, as they were leaving for PanChiao, they met Major Hwang with 5,000 soldiers. Good peaches were available at PanChiao. The next night they journeyed to ChangTi, each day traveling about 60 li, or 20 miles.

On August 14 a soldier escort sent to meet them held them back an hour. That day two coolies died from the heat and strenuous climb. Arriving at HwangTsoPa, they camped in the temple and called on the yamen (office or residence of a public official) in the evening. They spent a day resting at this camp and ate that evening at the yamen as guests of YuanChiang. The next day they proceeded to KaoTsen for the night. Here Lois and Julian found a big cave below waterfalls and took a refreshing swim, exploring the cave into which the stream flowed under the hill.

The next day, after a two hour delay at noon when their coolies ran away, they traveled 75 li to HsiaoYiCheng. Hiring three new coolies, they continued their journey and were met by an honor guard on the outskirts of HsiaoYiCheng, where they were all housed in the yamen and given a big dinner in the evening. The magistrate also insisted on giving them breakfast the next morning before they continued their journey to PaLin. The air was good and pink crape myrtle bloomed profusely in the temple yard where they stopped for the night. Lois held clinic in the evening and 20 or more persons came for medical treatment.

By August 27 they received mail from Yunnanfu and left Chin Cheng for Kweiyang, where the Governor and staff met them five li out of the city. After tea with the Governor of Kweichow province, they rode in his new Hudson automobile to the city's west gate. The automobile had been brought in pieces over the mountains by horseback and put together in Kweiyang for the pleasure and use of the Governor in this remote capitol city. A honeymoon cottage had been built to house O. J. Todd and his bride, Dr. Lois, in the Public Gardens at the center of the city. They were treated royally with the Governor entertaining them daily. The Governor was cordial and ordered a formal reception for them by the local Famine Relief Committee. Formal group photographs were taken and meetings were set with local engineers and commissioners. The Governor gave a theatre party in their honor on August 30 which lasted from 3:00 PM to 8:00 PM and included seeing 13 plays and eating a foreign style dinner! A band played marches between the plays. There were 52 invited guests.

On August 31 Lois, Julian, and companions went to ChienMing Shan on a picnic. Lois rode her horse up the stone steps to the top of the hill. Lois and her husband climbed to the top of the peak and took photos of Kweiyang. Julian attended the graduation exercises at the Cadet School the next day, accompanying the Governor to inspect the graduating cadets. On September 3 the Governor had flags up along the main street in honor of Engineer Todd and his bride and hosted a formal dinner followed by the Governor's official welcome speech.

On September 4, Lois and Julian arranged for two army mules for the rigorous trip north to Tsunyi, taking Chen, two mafoos, two guards and four coolies. Another 14 soldiers also went as a guard of honor. They traveled 70 li to TanTsao and another 70 li the next day to Sifeng. On September 6 they traveled 96 li, passing through valleys during rice harvest. Next day they traveled through farm land where workers were harvesting corn and beans, dropping from 2,500 feet elevation to 1,700 feet in 30 minutes. After crossing WuChang Ho (river), they climbed back up to 2,800 feet elevation, going 75 li that day. After 65 li on new road the next day, they arrived at Tsunyi, where they called on the magistrate. They spent the next two days in Tsunyi sightseeing. All the coolies left. The third day Julian walked 65 to 70 li on the new road and made tests of road grades with a hand level, finding 20 percent and 30 percent pitches. The fourth day he reported to the magistrate on his engineering consultation and made his recommendations on the road work.

Three new coolies were hired to carry the baggage and on September 13 they left Tsunyi with the magistrate seeing them off at the South Gate. A rigorous four day trip on mule back returned the couple to Kweiyang. They arrived late in the afternoon on September 16 at their comfortable honeymoon cottage in Kweiyang Public Gardens.

The next four days were spent resting and writing reports for the Governor of Kweichow and writing letters. More official luncheons followed, along with a dinner at the Governor's house on September 18. The Governor was very impressed with Dr. Lois's stamina and courage in undertaking this rigorous and dangerous journey by horseback. Lois was the first white woman to travel in this region. On September 20 they were invited again to have supper with the Governor and his wife. In the evening he gave them silk fabric, oiled silk (waterproofed with tung oil), and $200 cash in silver dollars as a wedding present.

On September 21 they rose early and left Kweiyang after an official farewell, a final ride in the Governor's Hudson automobile, and taking a photo of the Governor in his auto. Four new coolies had been hired for the journey to Anshen.

After traveling four days in rain on slippery roads, they reached Chenning with an escort of 13 soldiers. Lois helped at the hospital that evening. The next day there was no rain and they enjoyed some good persimmons at HwangKuSsu. They traveled through PaLinChiao canyon and photographed the stone bridge there, arriving at KwanLin by evening. The same 26 soldiers that escorted them the previous day continued with them on September 26 to MuYu where the magistrate sent them presents of pears, walnuts, and chestnuts. The next day rain made the roads muddy and the stone steps slippery. From MuYu they dropped 2,300 feet in less than three hours on a slippery trail, then climbed 1,700 feet in altitude to ChinMenKu and 600 more feet to PingKai where they stopped for the night. The next day they went 88 li on good roads to PaLin at an altitude of 4,000 feet and stopped at a temple for the night.

On September 29 they traveled 50 li to ShengJanHsien by noon and went to the yamen. Magistrate Lan put them up in his home. They visited the public gardens on a wooded hill where a temple was being built as a memorial to Governor Chou. Leaving in light rain the next morning, they went 75 li to WangTun, admiring many chestnut and walnut trees along the road. The next day they traveled 65 li to HwangTsoPa by 2:00 PM and were welcomed at the pagoda temple, where they were given the top room. The coolies asked to be released, but they refused to let them go. General Chang called on Lois and Julian and they returned his call; then they called on the magistrate. The next day they went 55 li to ChangTi and camped in a temple on a hill overlooking the bridge, but they got fleas from the room where they stayed. After a good horseback trip of 70 li the next day, they arrived at Pan Chiao at an altitude of 4,800 feet and occupied a loft in the barn of the same small farm where they had stopped in August.

The next morning they went 55 li to Lo Ping, called on Commander Lin and changed guard of 26 men, then went another 20 li to the foot of the valley to Chin Da Lo where they camped for the night at the new temple. After riding horseback 45 li to Tien Shan by noon the next morning, they ate and changed guards. Then went 40 more li to Shih Chang Hsien where they saw Colonel Huang and stayed in the old temple for the night. This day's trip on October 5 was 85 li and Julian walked over half the way, riding horseback the rest.

The trip from Shih Chang Hsien the next day to Ma Kai was 75 li. One coolie was left behind because of sickness. The magistrate sent one man with a letter to the Lu Liang magistrate to accompany them on October 6. They used no soldiers for escort that day. At Ma Kai they called on General Lo. The next morning they received word that the LuLiang magistrate would send them on if they went there. So they started out with General Lo's deputy, but rumors of bandit troops frightened him back to Ma Kai. They changed roads and went to Tai Peng Shao 35 li from Ma Kai and stayed in a farm house for the night. Chen quit the group when they started for Lu Liang. Yunnan troops went past in the night to LuLiang.

On October 8 they went to Tien Sheng Kwan by noon and after lunch went another 40 li to Pa Hsiao to stop for the night at the temple. The only soldiers they met that day were three or four at noon. The altimeter stayed between 5,400 and 5,600 feet elevation all day. The next morning was foggy but they went 35 li to ILiang before noon and the coolies and horse were fine. They reached a high point of 5,800 feet, then dropped to 4,400 feet at ILiang. At 2:00 PM Lois and her husband took the train to Yunnanfu, arriving at 5:00 PM on October 9.

They had left Yunnanfu by horseback for Kweichow on August 6, more than two months earlier. It had been quite a journey, both physically strenuous and full of risk and adventure.

In Yunnanfu they got their mail and stored baggage from the Consulate, went to a reception at the Governor's yamen, met with General Yung, met with the British Consul, French Consul, saw several missionaries, and met with U.S. Vice Consul Hagen. There were ten days of meetings, including the Famine Relief Committee, writing reports and letters and attending official functions.

On October 13 fighting just west of Yunnanfu resulted in a cut-off of lights and water. Four wounded soldiers were brought into Dr. Watson's hospital from the battle scene. On October 18 Lois and her husband went horseback riding and went to Ta Pan Chiao to review road work where 250 men were doing earthwork and 30 men were in quarries cutting stone for the project. The next day they went by horseback to visit the Confucian temple in the morning and the Copper Temple in the afternoon.

Lois and Julian left Yunnanfu by train on October 20 for Amichu. The next day their first class train compartment was taken over by soldiers, so Lois and Julian rode in a special train car with Mr. O'Kelly from Amichu to Lokay. The next day they continued by train to Hanoi and traveled that evening to Haifong.

In Haifong on October 23 they reservated space on the boat *San Po*, rested, bought lace and linen, and called on friends. They boarded the boat the next morning for the journey north, reaching Haikow at 10:00 AM October 25, spending the rest of the day at anchor discharging 80 tons of cargo and taking aboard 50 to 60 Chinese and a herd of pigs. The next morning the boat pulled anchor and sailed from Haikow to Hongkong, arriving October 27.

Next day they made reservations on the boat *Magnolia* to sail for Dairen, arriving in Shanghai on October 31; they continued on the *Magnolia* to Dairen, arriving November 3. Next morning they purchased tickets to sail from Dairen to Tientsin on the *Saitsu Maru*. All six cabins on the boat were full. Time on board was spent reading and writing letters. In the evening Lois played her Spanish guitar and sang ballads and American folk songs.

Arriving in Tientsin on the afternoon of November 5, they went by train the following day to Peking, where they would establish their home. It had been quite a honeymoon and wedding trip—over four months of arduous travel with danger and challenge, camping in primitive places, and a generous amount of adventure, traveling by horseback in remote, mountainous Kweichow province, China.

CHAPTER 6

Family in Peking

Peking (Beijing) was an ancient walled city, bustling and throbbing, in the 1920's and 1930's when Lois and her family made it their home. During the years when this beautiful, historic city served as China's capital it was called Peking or Beijing, which literally means northern capital. The nation's capital was moved south temporarily during war years to Nanking or Nanjing, which literally means southern capital. During this time the city's name was changed from Peking to Peiping, meaning northern peace.

In the 1920's and 1930's streets in Peking were unpaved, dusty and muddy, with open sewers or drainage ditches along the sides. Major intersections were marked by large, ornately painted wooden archways called Pai Lo's. They rose across the four approaches to the intersection: red enameled wooden columns, spread at a bracing angle, supported the carved wooden frieze which crossed over the street, topped by a green tiled roof, forming a decorative grid at major intersections.

Beneath these archways, along the crowded roads, men pulled rickshas transporting passengers. Wooden carts pulled by men, horses, donkeys or mules were used to transport cargo. Camel trains bringing fuel into the city were nearly a daily sight. Bactrim camels, with bags of coal slung between the humps on their backs, were roped together to form a long train or procession. They crossed the vast Gobi desert bringing coal from mountains in the far west to the capital. Automobiles and trucks were rare.

Street vendors and little shops crowded every street and alley (hutong). The aroma of herbs, spices, butcher shops, and street cafes filled the air. In winter the vendors roasted chestnuts and sweet potatoes over charcoal cauldrons on the street corners; steamed dumplings, noodles, and soup were always available along the streets. In summer the vendors sold glazed crabapples on wooden skewers (t'ang huler) as well as noodles, steamed dumplings, and other delicacies.

Musical sounds filled the air from vendors calling out their wares, squeaking wooden carts, beasts of burden, and pigeons with whistles attached to their tails (sometimes several whistles creating a musical chord when the bird flew through the air). Street urchins screamed out to passing foreigners in their rickshaws, "Dirty foreign devil" and spat upon them.

The stench of raw sewage in "honey pots" by the front doors along the streets was reinforced by the droppings from the beasts of burden used for transportation.

Lois and Julian spent the second week of November, 1927 in Peking house-hunting and started looking for furniture. They received word that the Gamble's House at the American Board Mission would be available the next week as the Gamble's would be on furlough. They bought some furniture from Dr. Wood, took their trunks out of storage, opened a bank account, and went shopping for other items needed for establishing their first home in Peking.

By November 10 the dysentery Julian acquired during their trip to Kweichow was getting worse. He was hospitalized for treatment at P.U.M.C. (Peking Union Medical College) on November 12. On November 20 he was also given medication for ascaris (roundworm). His weight had dropped from 165 to 143 pounds. The next day he was able to move into their new home and to start doing a little office work at home; within a few days he was going to his office for a few hours to write reports and resuming his busy work schedule. Lois was busy unpacking and furnishing their rented home. She was pregnant and expecting their first child in March, 1928.

By November 30 Julian was getting ready for a trip south to Shantung. Lois went along to Tehchow where she was met by Dr. Parsons and Alice Reed. She enjoyed the reunion with her former colleagues at the mission station. Julian went on to Tsinanfu to review the Red Cross work in Shantung and to hold meetings to assess the need for further famine relief work. From there his itinerary included Shanghai, Nanking, Wuhu, Kiukiang, Nanchang, and Fuchow. He returned home to Peking on December 24, just in time for Christmas at home with Lois.

They had a fine Christmas Day in Peking, going ice skating in the morning, going to the Christmas Service at Union Church in the afternoon, and having dinner guests at their home in the evening. Lois's gift to her husband was a camel hair comforter for his bed. Julian gave Lois a sable coat. The next day they went ice skating at P.U.M.C., read, and called on friends. It snowed that evening. Winters in Peking are cold and windy with light and infrequent snows, a six inch snowfall being unusually heavy. The temperature however can drop to three below zero; the chill factor is extreme.

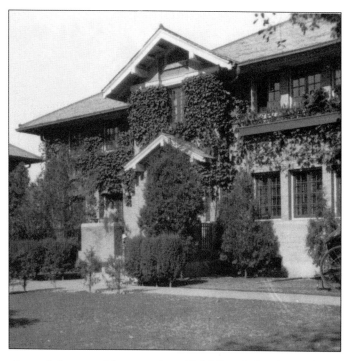

One of the rental homes where Todd family lived in Peking.

Dust storms begin in January, blowing out of the Gobi desert in the northwest, turning the air yellow and usually lasting five to ten minutes. Dust storms recur periodically through the winter and spring until the rainy season comes to settle the dry soil. Julian's work pattern, being gone from home a month or two at a time in the field on his engineering projects, then returning home to Peking and to his Famine Relief Commission office for a week or so to write reports and order supplies, continued from 1927 to 1938. Lois's independence and self-sufficiency in managing their household and raising their family grew during her husband's long periods away. Her strength, stamina, courage, and commitment to her family, her medical profession, and her Christian calling were remarkable.

Lois and Julian's social activities in Peking included daily ice skating in winter on the frozen, flooded tennis courts at P.U.M.C., the Peking Club, or on the frozen lake at Pei Hai (Winter Park) north of the Forbidden City, bowling at the Peking Club, dancing at the Peking Hotel, attending and giving dinner parties in their home for twelve to twenty guests, attending concerts and theater performances. Most of their social activities were shared with their close friends from the American Board (Kung Li Hui), Lois's colleagues from her years as as a medical missionary in Tehchow. There were also afternoon teas, house guests, outings with the ladies of the American Board, and occasionally a movie.

Julian, in addition to his extended periods of time away from home, established the Shantung Mint Company to raise peppermint in north China.

This was a hobby, stemming from his own childhood experience of helping his father and his uncle, Albert Todd, raise mint on the farm near Kalamazoo, Michigan. This experiment in Shantung province was successful and eventually led to the production of mint wafers which were packed in tins for sale or for gifts. These mints became a favorite gift for their friends and their household servants at Christmas time in Peking. Julian also established a peppermint garden, or small farm, near Peking which he visited often when he was at home.

Lois provided medical care to the missionaries with Kung Li Hui in Peking and also to other Americans in Peking. She also did some clinical teaching at Peking Union Medical College (Rockefeller Foundation Medical Center) in Peking. She wrote and published a paper on toxoplasmosis, a clinical report on several cases she had diagnosed and treated in Tehchow.

In addition to serving as attending physician to American Board personnel and clinical teaching at Peking Union Medical College, she worked at the Presbyterian Hospital. Later, when her children began attending Peking American School, she became the school physician with regular office hours at the school.

Julian spent time reading books as well as writing technical engineering reports, articles for the "National Geographic Magazine" and for engineering journals. Later during their China years Julian wrote two books, one about his 20 year career devoted to harnessing the Yellow River, entitled *Two Decades in China*, and the other one about his collection of ancient Chinese bronze mirrors, entitled *Chinese Bronze Mirrors* (co-athored by Milan Rupert).

Much of his time was devoted to meetings with officials in various agencies as well as government and the military in order to assure permission and cooperation for his engineering projects (including famine relief, flood control, and reconstruction of the Grand Canal).

Julian actively participated in the Scottish Rite Lodge of Peking, taking a leadership role whenever he was home. He was also an active participant in the Michigan Club, an association of both Chinese and Caucasian alumni from University of Michigan.

Julian's main responsibilities as chief engineer for the Famine Relief Commission of China included flood control of the Yellow River ("China's Sorrow") and reconstruction of the Grand Canal. Connecting north China with south China, the Grand Canal was first built during the Chou dynasty, 200 B.C. He frequently had emergency trips by train from Peking to the site of breaks in the dikes that contained the Yellow River.

One such trip in March 1928 took him by train to Tsinanfu, then by Dodge car all day to the breaks in the south dike of the Yellow River, five miles below Li Chin. Ice was eight to ten feet high on the mud flats in the river. Hundreds of refugees were building huts in the dike. He had to relocate the refugees, recruit laborers, and bring in rock fill from an old fill in an obsolete section of dike to repair the breaks in the new dike. Building new channels for the Yellow River and diverting the river into these channels was an important part of his engineering work in addition to repairing breaks in the dikes.

On March 16, 1928, Lois was admitted to P.U.M.C. for observation due to eclampsia. Their first baby was due in a week. Julian received a cable from

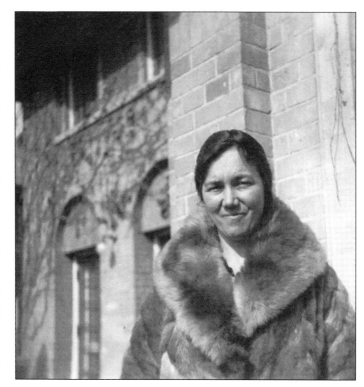

Lois in her sable coat, Peking.

J. E. Baker regarding a famine emergency at Lintsing in Shantung and another from Engineer Wong at Kweichow regarding 200,000 men at work on roads. On March 18 Julian left for Lintsing but found the Yellow River Bureau had delayed its negotiations, so returned to Peking on March 22, arriving at P.U.M.C. just a few hours before Lois gave birth to Doris Jean. Lois and her baby, Doris, were still hospitalized at P.U.M.C. when Julian left Peking on March 29 to take care of Shantung famine matters. He returned to Peking on April 5 and took Lois and baby home from the hospital on April 6, 1928.

Lois and Julian enjoyed going for long walks together in Peking. One of their favorite outings was to walk along the parkway on top of the city wall behind the Legation district. Another was climbing Coal Hill, north of the Forbidden City in central Peking, or walking in Pei Hai, just west of Coal Hill. Summer Palace, northwest on the outskirts of Peking, was another favorite place to walk.

On April 14, Lois's birthday, a lovely warm spring day, they celebrated by going out for some ice cream (a rare treat in a land where dairy products usually were not available). Julian bought some fresh flowers for Lois and composed special verses in honor of the occasion. He composed sets of verses for every birthday, anniversary, and holiday for the family from then until Lois's death 40 years later. He also wrote verses about special journeys and experiences.

In May and through the summer Lois and Julian played tennis nearly every evening at the Peking Club or at P.U.M.C., as it was too hot during the day to participate in strenuous activity. When Julian was away on his business trips, Lois played tennis with Laura Cross and other friends from Kung Li Hui.

FURLOUGH TO AMERICA

In June 1928 Lois, Julian, and baby Doris left Peking for a visit to U.S.A. to see their families. Departure from Peking to Tientsin by auto was difficult with vehicles stuck in the muddy, rutted roads and soldiers stopping autos and holding them for ransom. Julian's hired auto was the only one to get through. They gathered their baggage in Tientsin and sailed for Japan, Hawaii and U.S.A. Baby Doris travelled in a woven basket which also served as her bassinet.

Arriving in Seattle four weeks after leaving Peking, they enjoyed a family reunion in Eugene, Oregon, at the home of Julian's sister Vera. Their parents, Julia and Oliver Hovey Todd, were present as were Victor (Julian's oldest brother) and Donna (Julian's youngest sister).

The two week visit at Vera's home included trips up the McKenzie River to the Cliff Trail above Belknap Springs, to Salem and Corvallis, Klamath Falls, Crater Lake, and the top of Mt. Garfield. From Eugene they travelled by train to San Francisco and Oakland to visit Walter (Julian's younger brother) and his wife Ida, as well as sister Donna and John McBryan, friends from Lois' university days in Berkeley, and friends from Julian's engineering days in San Francisco.

Morris and Gladys Pendleton arrived from Los Angeles and took Lois, Julian, and baby Doris to Saratoga to see the Pendleton family home and prune ranch on Farwell Avenue, where Lois grew up, and to visit family relatives in the vicinity, including trips to Santa Cruz and Capitola, Big Basin Redwood Park, and the beloved mountain place, Minnewawa, above Saratoga. They also enjoyed traveling by car to Lake Tahoe, Fallen Leaf, Yosemite and Tuolumne Meadows, Tioga Pass and Mono Lake, then Mirror Lake, and via Merced to Gilroy, Watsonville, and Monterey. They continued by car south along the Pacific coast through Paso Robles and Santa Barbara to San Gabriel and Morris and Gladys' home. Visits with Lois's mother, Jessie, Grandmother Adaline, and eleven year old sister Adaline, plus calls on many missionary friends living at Pilgrim Place in Claremont, filled the next week.

In mid-August Lois, Julian, and baby Doris took the train east via Ogden and Cheyenne to Denver, where they were met by Julian's brother Alfred Todd and his daughter Priscilla and taken to their home in Lamar, in southeastern Colorado near the Kansas border. It was 100 degrees in Alf's home at noon

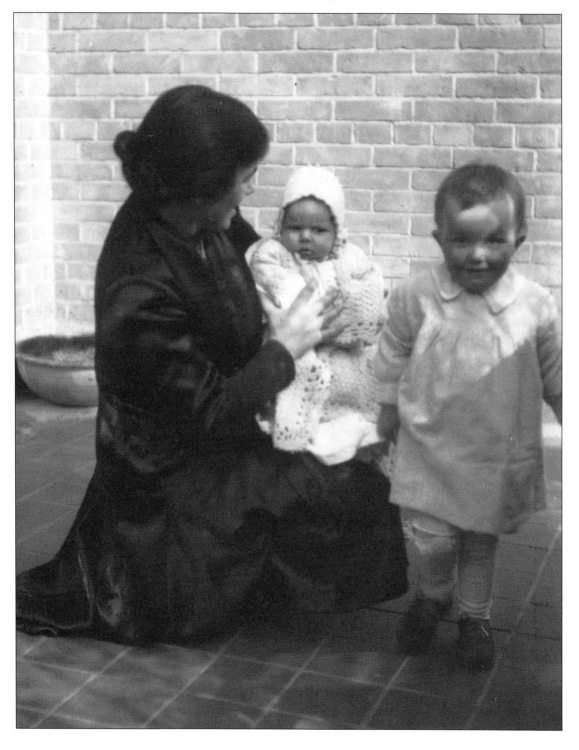

Lois holding Elinor at 3 months with Doris at 23 months in Peking, 1930.

in mid-August. Of course air-conditioning was not available in those days. After a week in Lamar, they continued by train to Chicago and Kalamazoo, Michigan, where Julian had spent his high school years. They visited Nottowa and the old Farrand home where Julian's mother had been raised, and Colon where Julian was born, and visited his Uncle Albert's two mint farms and distilleries near Campania.

After a week in southern Michigan they continued east by train to Ann Arbor, Detroit, and New York. After several days in New York and in Boston on business in early September, they took a night boat from Boston to Belfast, Maine, to visit Pendleton cousins and aunts in Belfast and Searsport, Maine. Lois and Doris spent a week in Rockland, Maine, with friends. Julian went to New York to spend six weeks on business with China Famine Relief, American Society of Civil Engineers, and China Society. There were also trips to Washington, D.C., to visit Julian's brother Laurence Todd, a journalist.

In November they took the train from New York to Seattle via Detroit, Ann Arbor, and Kalamazoo with a stop in Minneapolis to visit Lois's cousins. Another week was spent in Eugene with Vera for shopping and packing for the return ocean voyage to China. Lois, Julian, and baby Doris left from San Francisco by ship on November 23, 1928 arriving in Yokohama on December 10 with a three day stop with friends in Kobe. They arrived at Taku Bar and Tientsin on December 17 and took the train to Peking the next day.

RESUMING LIFE IN PEKING

During the six month furlough to America, Lois and Julian had left their household furnishings stored in the attic at the Shaw's home, as the house they had leased was needed to house another American family. Another house was found for Lois and Julian and they moved their things from the attic of Beth and Ernest Shaw's home and proceeded to get settled in their new home. On Christmas Day there was a Christmas tree for Doris. Lois and Julian went ice skating in the forenoon at Peking Club and played deck tennis in the afternoon on the Shaw's back yard tennis court after church.

After the six months abroad, Lois interviewed and hired a new amah (live-in babysitter) to care for Doris and a new cook and a houseboy. Since she was a physician, Lois required all applicants for any domestic job in her household to provide a full medical history and a recent chest x-ray to rule out active tuberculosis, in addition to a personal interview.

In April when Julian was home in Peking, between his lengthy field trips to work on the Yellow River, he made a garden and planted lettuce for the family's table use. Lois enjoyed raising flowers. She knew all flowers, shrubs, and

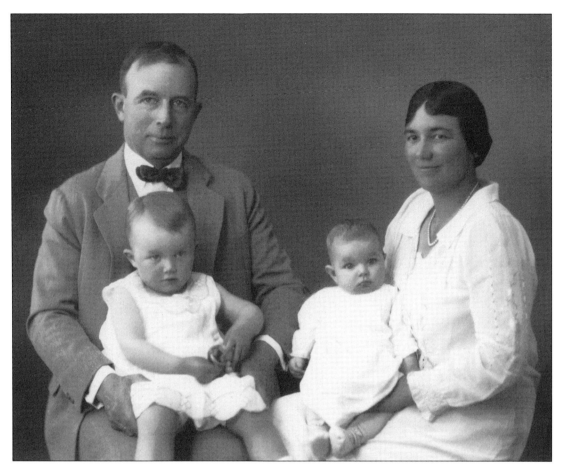

Todd family in Peking, 1930: O. J. Todd with Doris and Lois with Elinor.

trees by their botanical as well as common names, having grown up with her older brother, Robert, who was an avid botany student.

Tennis games and deck tennis were favorite social activities when winter was over and outdoor ice skating was no longer possible. Occasional movies were shown in Peking to add variety to the indoor evening activities of bowling and ballroom dancing, so popular in Peking at that time. Dinner parties at home continued to be popular and were easy to accomplish with ample domestic help. These dinner parties were often formal and included from ten to twenty guests.

Although domestic help was readily available, no household appliances were available. Laundry was done by hand by a full-time laundry man who washed all the linens, bedding and clothing by hand in a washtub with a washboard, hung them on a line to dry, and then sprinkled and ironed every item by hand with an iron heated on the coal stove. Fresh vegetables, fruits, meat, poultry or fish were purchased by the cook daily. Food was stored in a pantry. Canned butter, which was often rancid, came by ship from Australia and canned powdered milk, "Klim", came from America. The cook prepared the meals on a large cast iron stove which burned coal briquets. Running the household required the efforts of a minimum of four servants: laundry man, cook, house boy (dishwashing and house-cleaning), and ricksha man providing transportation (children to school, cook to market, and adults to work, shopping, recreation). If you had children, a live-in amah for child-care and a sewing girl to make clothes (from underwear to coats) also were needed.

Each summer in June most of the Americans in north China took their families by train to Pei Tai Ho, the beach resort on the Yellow Sea one hundred eighty miles due east of Peking, for two or three months. Summers in Peking were extremely hot and difficult to tolerate, especially for children. At Pei Tai Ho the nights were cool and there were fine swimming beaches. After getting their families settled for the summer at Pei Tai Ho, the men usually returned to Peking for another four to six weeks of work before going to the beach for a holiday with their families and to bring them home. Recreation at Pei Tai Ho included playing tennis on clay courts and swimming in the ocean each morning and afternoon. Lois made daily medical rounds riding a donkey, carrying her black medical bag to make house calls on American Board families needing medical care.

Lois won the ladies doubles tennis tournament in August 1929 while pregnant with her second child, Elinor, born three months later in November. Baseball games, donkey polo races, picnics, and military band concerts added variety to the summer activities. Night swims when the ocean was phosphorescent were a special treat. Daytime excursions and picnics by donkey to the sand dunes north of Pei Tai Ho were fun. Some favorite places for picnics were Lotus Hills, Eagle Rock, and Lighthouse Point. When the Todd children were older, the family enjoyed an all day outing by train to ShanHaiKuan to the north; donkeys were hired at the train station for the ride up the mountain to the temple which had a spectacular view of the Great Wall meeting the sea.

In August 1929 Lois and Julian moved to a house in the South Compound of Peking Union Medical College. This continued to be their home for several years. When their second child, Lois Elinor, was born, Julian was in Peking a week prior to the birth and two weeks following the birth for report writing, meetings, and entertaining visiting engineers. Julian brought Lois and baby Elinor home from P.U.M.C. at nine days and left a few days later for field work at Saratsi (where all the missionaries had recently died of typhus). He returned to Peking in mid-December and stayed at home through Christmas, writing reports on the Saratsi work.

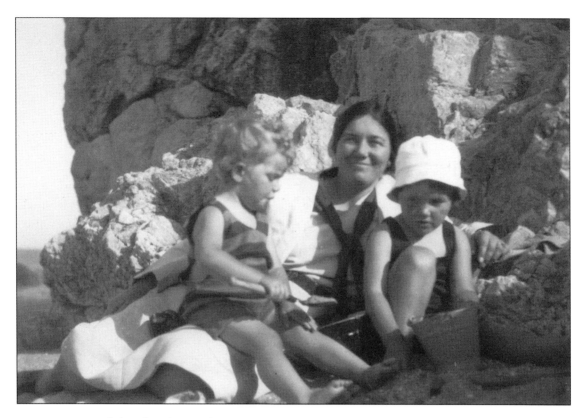

Lois with her daughters, Elinor and Doris, at the beach, Pei Tai Ho, July 1931.

In January 1930 Lois and Julian resumed their daily ice skating and began taking Doris, age 22 months, for walks on the city wall. By March when the ice skating season ended, Lois and Julian played tennis daily, as weather permitted, unless he was away on field work.

Julian was installed as Wise Master in Scottish Rite in Peking in June 1930 before taking Lois and babies to Pei Tai Ho for the summer. After a few days at the seashore, enjoying swimming, tennis, and fresh strawberry shortcake, Julian returned to Peking to complete errands. Then he went by train to Saratsi, where he directed a river diversion Intake project. The work was badly complicated by bandit raids, murders, rainy weather, and supply shortages. Coolies (laborers) were paid in grain (millet or wheat) for their work in stone quarries, gravel pits, cement work, building stone dikes and bridges, driving piles and moving earth, either in baskets balanced upon poles over their shoulders or in Chinese wooden wheelbarrows and carts. Traditional wooden Chinese wheelbarrows are much easier to push than Western wheelbarrows since the wheel is under the center of the wheelbarrow and thus carries the weight of the load.

In August 1930 Lois won the ladies singles tennis tournament for North China at Pei Tai Ho. Doris was 29 months old and Elinor, still nursing, was eight months. Lois's tennis victory ended the summer fun. An influx of jelly fish in August made swimming at the seashore so hazardous that the family returned early to Peking.

Little Doris was hospitalized at P.U.M.C. in September with a high fever. Lois sent a wire to Julian in Saratsi asking him to come home. He arrived two days later. Lois stayed with Doris night and day at the hospital for several days. Exhausted by the fourth night, Lois hired a special nurse to stay with Doris. A week later Doris was improved and came home from the hospital on the ninth day.

Julian returned to his field work in Saratsi a few days later. In Saratsi 60 tons of cement were unloaded from trains for making concrete blocks for construction of the head gates. But bandit activity forced Julian to return to Peking after only three weeks in the field. Always restless, he began plans for a trip to Sian.

In November, Julian came home to Peking for Elinor's first birthday, celebrated with a party, and for Thanksgiving, then off to Shanghai to market his peppermint oil and to purchase some mint machinery. He returned to Peking in mid-December and remained at home through January.

Dr. Edward F. Parsons, a capable physician who worked with Lois at the mission hospital in Tehchow, was hospitalized at P.U.M.C. with influenza and pneumonia and died March 8, 1931, at the age of 34 in the prime of life. Graduated from University of Michigan Medical School in 1922, he did special post-graduate study in psychiatry before going to China in 1925 as a missionary doctor. He worked at Williams-Porter Hospitals in Tehchow until 1928, when he was transferred to Tunghsien to take charge of the mission hospital. His death was a terrible loss to the American Board and all his colleagues in China.

Helping to soften the loss a bit, Julian purchased two beautiful ebony and rosewood chests with tinted, carved ivory flowers and birds for Lois for her birthday. They came from the imperial household. He left for Saratsi again a week before her birthday, as staff and supplies had been gathered to continue the project. Two weeks later he was back home in Peking for seven days then returned to Saratsi with a mason and a carpenter. By May there were 2,000 soldiers helping to dig the new canal for the Yellow River.

When Julian returned from his fieldwork in June, Elinor at age 19 months was hospitalized at P.U.M.C. with dysentery. Lois gave up the house and stayed with friends, Steve and Lethe Pyle. Julian boarded a train back to Saratsi five days later because 1,000 more soldiers had just arrived to help excavate the

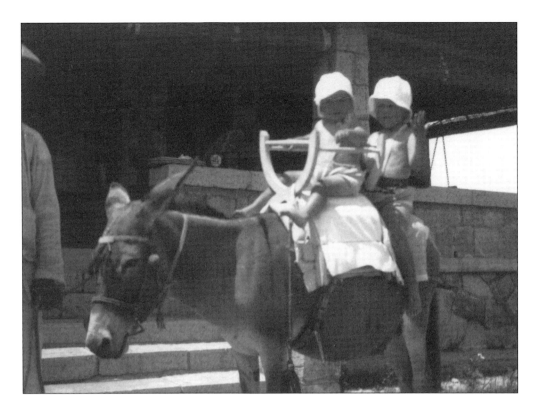

Elinor and Doris riding their donkey to the beach, Pei Tai Ho, 1931.

new canal near the Intake. Robert Pendleton, older brother of Lois, had come from the Philippines to China to do soils studies, see the Saratsi project, and conduct a soil survey. He was present with various dignitaries from Peking for the dedication ceremonies on June 22, 1931.

The Peking Zoological Garden, west of the city, became a favorite outing for the Todd children. The zoo's two gatekeepers were brothers and true giants, each seven to eight feet tall. When little, the Todd children looked up to the giants' knees with awe and amazement. Among the freak animals living at the zoo were a cyclops pig with one eye in the middle of its forehead and a cow with five hooves—one at the end of its tail, rather hazardous when swatting flies.

The Temple of Heaven, on the southeast outskirts of Peking, was another favorite place to visit with the beautiful royal blue glazed tile roofs, semicircular "whispering wall", and spacious, tiered marble altar. As the family grew, the children came along on these outings, in a baby carriage at first until they were ready to walk, and then by foot. As the children grew older there were hikes and picnics in the Western Hills, west of Peking, as well as weekend outings to the various parks in and around Peking.

On July 1 Lois and Julian went to Pei Tai Ho with their two little girls and rented a beach house at East Cliff. Lois was very careful in protecting her children from excessive sun exposure, allowing them to be in the sun only 15 minutes the first day, 20 the next day, and 25 the following day, gradually working up to an hour or so at a time, to prevent sunburn and to build up golden tans. When outside the children always had to wear white broad brimmed cotton hats (with elastic straps under the chin) to prevent heat stroke.

July 2, their fourth wedding anniversary, was celebrated with a dinner party at the beach house for six guests. Mrs. Pyle and Alice Reed stayed for the month of July as house guests. In addition to morning and afternoon swims, Lois and Julian usually played two or three sets of tennis on the clay courts each morning, and another two or three sets in the afternoon when it wasn't raining. After three weeks, Julian took the train to Peking and made business trips to Tientsin and to the project at Saratsi. In mid-August he returned by train to Pei Tai Ho to be with the family and to take them home to Peking.

Two days later Julian departed on a month long trip to Kansu. He spent five days at home in Peking for errands and correspondence and then was off to his field project at Saratsi for ten days, home for a day, then on the train for Shanghai and Nanking, back home to Peking in a week, and two days later off again on another field trip looking for a good dam site.

In mid-October Julian was back home in Peking and stayed writing reports and handling other business matters for three weeks. His birthday on November 1 was celebrated with a noon dinner party for ten, followed by photographing the children, Doris and Elinor. The next day he was on his way to Shanghai again, returning home three weeks later for Thanksgiving. Lois went to P.U.M.C. the next day for observation due to elevated blood pressure. A week later on December 5, 1931 their third child, James Pendleton, was born, weighing over 11 pounds. Lois and baby James came home from the hospital on the ninth day. Doris and Elinor were wild with joy over their baby brother. Christmas 1931 was beautiful with snow on the ground and a moonlight serenade of Christmas carols in the compound by the Salvation Army. Christmas morning the children delighted in a small decorated tree and several gifts to open. The day ended with a dinner party followed by home movies.

Julian spent January in Shanghai, Nanking, Wuhan, and environs of the Yangtze River on engineering business. After a few days at home in Peking he was off on field work again, spending most of February and March away. Lois kept herself busy at home in Peking raising their three small and lively children, doing some clinical teaching at P.U.M.C., and enjoying social and church activities with her friends of the American Board (Kung Li Hui).

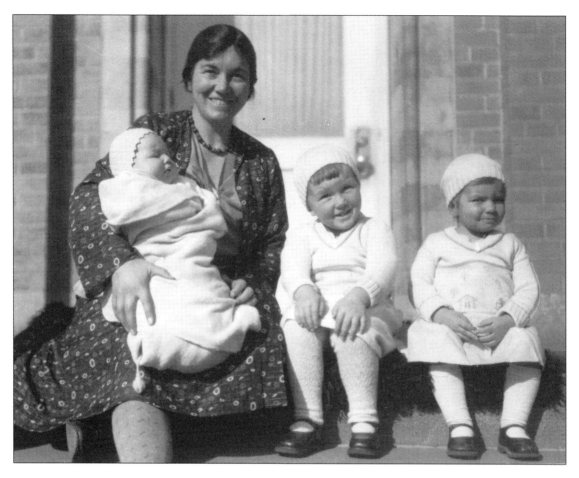

Lois with her children Feb. 1932: baby James, Doris nearly 4 and Elinor age 2.

FAMILY DEVOTIONALS

The Todd family gathered around the dining room table together three times a day for breakfast, lunch, and supper, beginning every meal with a blessing. When the children were little they sang together with their mother the morning blessing:

> "Father we thank Thee for the night
> And for the pleasant morning light,
> For rest and food and loving care,
> And all that makes the world so fair."

Later, as the children grew older, a second verse was added:

> "Help us to do the things we should,
> To be to others kind and good,
> In all we do in work or play,
> To grow more loving every day."

Every evening, after the children put on their nightgowns and brushed their teeth, Lois gathered the children around her in the nursery to sing songs together for 20 or 30 minutes before they went to bed. Sitting in her little wooden rocking chair, she played her Spanish guitar and taught them American folk songs, ballads, lullabies, sea chanties, and patriotic songs such as "My Country 'Tis of Thee" and "America the Beautiful," ending with "Goodnight Ladies" as the children skipped off to their beds.

Then Lois tucked each of her children into bed, saying with each one their evening prayer:

> "Now I lay me down to sleep.
> Guard me while in slumber deep.
> In the morn when I awake,
> Help me Lord, Thy way to take,
> For Jesus' sake. Amen.

A hug and kiss followed the prayer and then "Sweet dreams!"

DEAN OF CANTERBURY

At the end of April, Julian met Hewlett Johnson, the Dean of Canterbury at a luncheon at Dr. Maxwell's home in Peking. Dean Johnson accompanied Julian to Saratsi, where he and Lennig Sweet, Y.M.C.A. director of Peking, spent the month of May traveling with Julian in the interior of China. They experienced many adventures including bandit raids, getting stuck in muddy and rutted roads, and being stopped by soldiers' gunfire. They visited curio shops while in the remote interior of China to shop for Chinese antiques for the Dean of Canterbury to take home to England.

PEI TAI HO

During Julian's absence, Lois moved to a house in the North Compound of P.U.M.C. When Julian returned from his travels, the family took the train to Pei Tai Ho to spend the summer of 1932 at their beach house at East Cliff. Julian installed a flush toilet with a water tank and pull-chain high on the wall in their beach house, the first flush toilet in the community. Julian returned to Peking to resume his work in Saratsi and in Sian.

Alice Reed spent a month with Lois and the children in their East Cliff summer home at Pei Tai Ho. The lovely, lazy days at the seashore were filled with the children going by donkey to Baby Beach in the morning to play in the sand, wade, and paddle in the gently lapping waves, coming home for lunch and a nap, then returning to the beach for an afternoon swim. Lois enjoyed swimming with her children in addition to making medical rounds by donkey, and playing ten-

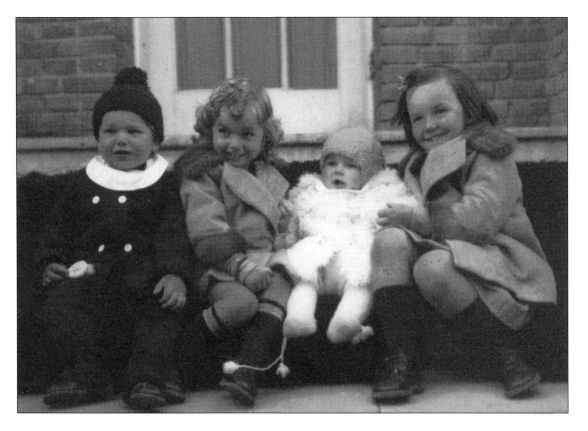

Todd children in Peking, November, 1933: James, Elinor, Hewlett, and Doris.

nis daily. Alice Reed swam, read books, wrote letters to her family, prepared lessons for her school at Techow, and knitted sweaters. The children loved going to Lotus Hill to see the deer and have a picnic. There were also picnics at Rocky Point, Eagle Rock, or Light House Point. For their trips to the beach Doris and Elinor shared one donkey, Elinor riding inside the wooden frame on the donkey's back and Doris holding on behind her. The summer days at Pei Tai Ho were pleasant, comfortable, and idyllic. Julian spent three weeks in July with his family, before going to Peking by train to resume his work in August, and returned to Pei Tai Ho for a few days the end of August to take his family back to Peking.

BACK IN PEKING

Robert Pendleton arrived from Nanking to take up residence in Lois and Julian's home in Peking. When Julian returned a few weeks later from field work, he and Lois took the girls to the newly opened Forbidden City for an outing in central Peking. In October 1932 Julian received word from Shansi that they wanted him to take charge of conservancy work there. Doris and Elinor hoped to celebrate their father's birthday with a party on November 1, but instead they went to the "flying field" to see him off in a European monoplane transporting him to Taiyuan.

By mid-November Julian was back in Peking. Elinor's third birthday was celebrated with a big party including a dozen children and seven ladies. Julian stayed in Peking working at his office for the next six weeks so he was home through both Thanksgiving and Christmas. Christmas was a big day in 1932 with Robert and Julian playing badminton at the Club after gifts had been opened, then dinner guests at 1 P.M., and an organ concert at the Peking Union Church at 5 P.M.

After Julian completed the Intake and diversion canal at Saratsi, the Saratsi Irrigation Association was formed to operate the new irrigation system that Julian and his staff built. In January 1933 when he visited the project in Saratsi again to be sure all was going well, it was eight below zero at 6:00 AM in Saratsi. He returned to Peking for a few days, greeted by shouts of joy from his three children, and enjoyed daily tennis and ice skating with Lois when at home. A few days later Julian was off to Pukow, Shanghai, Nanking (where foreign and Chinese gunboats were running all night), then Tientsin, and home to Peking two weeks later, after delays by troop trains, including cavalry going toward ShanHaiKwan.

The next month Julian was home with the family, ice skating daily with Lois, playing three or four sets of badminton daily with Robert at the Peking Club, writing reports and journal articles, scheduling many official meetings and social functions, and taking Lois, Doris, and Elinor on outings to Pei Hai lake or to Peking Club to ice skate. Doris and Elinor learned to ice skate by pushing straight-back chairs in front of them on the ice to acquire their balance. Soon they were skating between their parents, holding the hands of both parents, one on each side.

By mid-February Julian left for a month of field work in Shansi to survey the site for a new dam. When he returned home to Peking, he brought with him ornately painted black lacquered Shansi chests for Lois and for the girls. Doris and Elinor were delighted with the two small Shansi chests their father had brought for them; a place to store their treasures and to have doll tea parties.

A few days later he was off again for a week's trip to Pukow, Shanghai, and Nanking, returning home to Peking just in time to attend Scottish Rite Lodge, where he got a jewel as Past Wise Master, and to take Lois to P.U.M.C. in labor with their fourth child, Hewlett Freeman, who was born 36 hours later on March 19, 1933. Doris and Elinor were elated at the news of another baby brother. Doris became five years old on March 22. Lois and baby Hewlett came

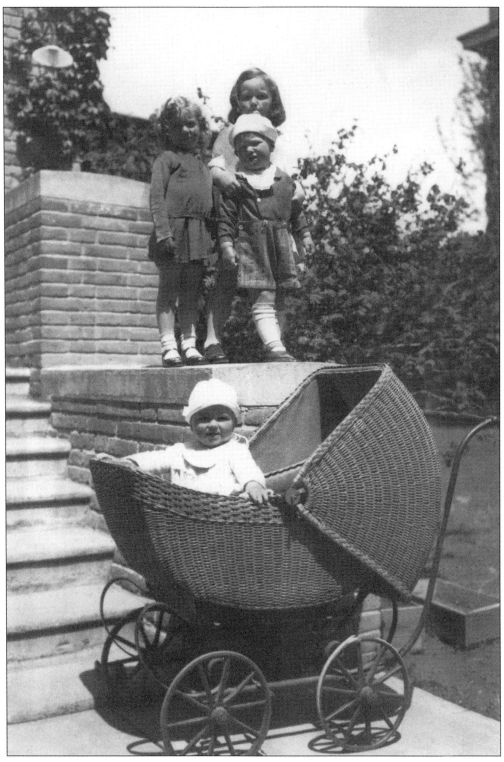

Todd children on front steps of their home at College of Chinese Studies, Peking, May 1934.

home from P.U.M.C. on the tenth day. The baby was named after Hewlett Johnson, Dean of Canterbury, who had traveled with Julian in China the previous year, and John R. Freeman, the San Francisco civil engineer who brought Julian to China in 1920.

While Julian was away in Shansi for the month of April, spring arrived in Peking with its beautiful flowering fruit trees in the sheltered gardens and parks, followed by lilacs and peonies in bloom with their heavenly fragrance. When Julian returned home from Shansi and Shensi in early May, he took Lois, Doris, and Elinor to PaoMaChang on the outskirts of Peking to see the horse races, to Shih-Lu project, and Paitechu. There were also trips with the children to the Temple of Heaven and to Yenching to see his peppermint farm, and a picnic supper at Pei Hai.

After a week at home Julian was off to Saratsi to look at breaks in four of the eight Laterals (irrigation canals) that had been completed two years earlier. From there he went west to Sian (now Xian), returning home to Peking the end of May to help Lois move the family to a new house at the Language School (College of Chinese Studies), a walled compound that included three private homes in addition to apartment buildings for married students, dormitories, dining halls, and classroom buildings. The Pettus family were the neighbors on one side and the Creighton family on the other side.

In early June Lois and Julian took the three oldest children for a walk up Coal Hill and to Pei Hai for a boat ride. James at 18 months was walking everywhere, even carrying a walking stick like his father.

After a week at home Julian was off to Taiyuan, using mules and horses for exploring the second dam site and the sulphur and coal mines in the region. He was home again three weeks later to write letters and reports and to do errands. The whole family enjoyed a picnic and outing to WuFooSsu, in the Western Hills outside Peking. Because Julian had to take the train to Chengchow and Sian in late June, the family did not go to Pei Tai Ho until mid-July. Alice Reed was in Peking with the family waiting to go with them to the beach. It was so very hot in Peking that the children's skin broke out with "prickly heat" and they were miserable. Lois had a barrel maker build a wooden swimming pool, about ten feet in diameter and sixteen inches deep, out of barrel half-staves to keep the children cool. The wooden swimming pool was built near the front entrance steps to the house, under the shade of a mulberry tree.

When the family arrived at Pei Tai Ho in mid-July with Alice Reed, it was a blessed relief to reach the cool sea breeze. The sea water was warm and clear for swimming. The family settled into their beach house and enjoyed the rest of the summer with its balmy days and pleasant activities.

Julian returned to Peking a few days later to resume his work, including trips to Taiyuan, Chengchow, and Sianfu. A month later he returned to Pei Tai Ho. He spent several days with tools and two coolies removing bad rocks from the beach below the house, doing most of the work with crow bar and sticks of dynamite in early morning at low tide.

At the end of each summer, he always took home on the train to Peking a large grain bag filled with clean beach sand. The sand was used with great care and pleasure by the Todd children for play in their large sand bowl on the porch. It had to last until the next summer. This year he filled six bags with clean beach sand to take to Peking for the Kindergarten at Peking American School, saving a bag of sand for the family's sand bowl, where his children played happily by the hour. In early September the family returned to Peking with their baggage plus the six bags of beach sand.

A few days later Julian was on his way by train to Shanghai, Nanking, Saratsi, and Taiyuan, returning home two weeks later to handle accounts, letters, reports, and errands. A week later he went to Chengchow and Sian for two weeks. After two days at home he took the railway to Nanking and Shanghai to purchase a new air compressor and air drills for the Yellow River job. The next month included many field trips.

PEKING AMERICAN SCHOOL

When the children were ready for school, Lois enrolled them at the Peking American School, a fine private school on the East side of Peking which included kindergarten through high school in one three story building (two stories plus basement). The students included about one third American, one third educated Chinese, and one third from various foreign embassies in Peking from most of the major nations of the world.

Miss Alice Moore was the principal and the curriculum was college preparatory, combining the best of the European curriculum and the American curriculum. For example, foreign languages were mandatory and introduced at an early age. Mandarin Chinese reading and writing were required beginning in the third grade. The children started French in the fourth or fifth grade and continued Chinese language reading and writing. Latin was started in the sixth or seventh grade and the two previous languages were continued. Spanish, German, Italian, and Russian were offered to the older children. By the time students graduated from high school they were fluent in several languages and also well schooled in geography, history, literature, mathmatics, and science.

Lois worked as school physician at Peking American School during the years her children attended the school, providing medical care and immunizations to all the children attending.

Julian was home in Peking the first week of November and enjoyed a dinner party for 14 guests which Lois had planned to celebrate his birthday. Three sets of tennis games were the daily routine when he was at home (usually from 4:45 to 5:30 PM), either singles with Lois or doubles if some of their friends could join them. Then he was off again to Shansi for the Water Conservancy Commission work on the No.2 dam and No.3 dam on the Yellow River. After ten days at his Taiyuan office, he returned to his Peking office for four days, then was off on a field trip to Saratsi for four days.

Julian was at home for Elinor's fourth birthday party and for Thanksgiving, then left for ten days in Sian and Chengchow. He purchased ancient Chinese bronzes, bronze mirrors, cups, and ceremonial vessels during each of his field trips, gradually adding to his collection. His collection of Chinese bronzes seemed like a wise investment during the depression years, when neither banks nor the stock market in the U.S. were safe, and it was difficult for foreigners to invest in real estate in China. He planned to eventually sell his collection of ancient Chinese bronzes to pay for his children's college educations in America.

The family regularly attended Sunday worship services at the P.U.M.C. Church or Peking Union Church, either at 11:00 AM or at 5:00 PM. After lunch they often went to Pei Hai, Temple of Heaven, Summer Palace, or the Peking Zoological Garden for an outing on Sunday afternoon.

Christmas 1933 was fully celebrated with both morning and 5:00 PM services on December 24, followed by Christmas caroling in the Language School compound by the Salvation Army. Christmas Day was great for the four children with gifts to open in the morning. Lois and Julian played two sets of tennis later. Guests came for dinner at 1:00 PM. The next day they went to a large Mission dinner at TungFu in the evening. And the following day three inches of snow fell.

Lois made a small Santa Claus costume that fit a six year old child and Doris, the eldest, played the role of Santa Claus by handing out Christmas gifts to family members on Christmas morning. Each Christmas thereafter, the child in the family who fit into the costume played the role of Santa Claus, distributing gifts to the family on Christmas morning.

Julian's returns home from field work were times of special joy and rejoicing. Lois was always relieved and happy to have her husband home again safe and sound. All the moments together were cherished. She was interested in his work and proud of his achievements. The children were exuberant to see their Daddy and eager to play and romp with him. Riding on his foot and singing "Bobby Shafto's Gone to Sea" was a favorite game as well as playing "Skin the Cat" (placing their hands between their legs and being flipped over by their father grasping their hands and pulling upward) and "Somersault" (grasping

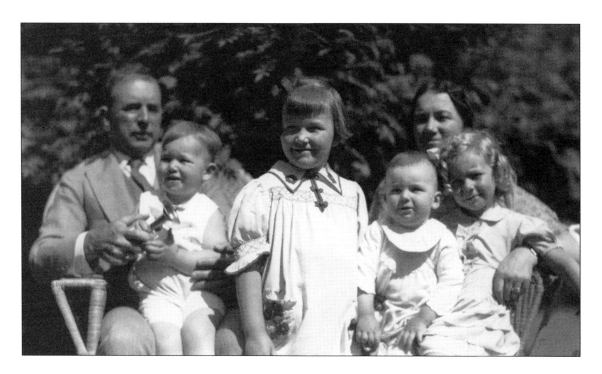

Todd family in Peking, Nov. 1934.

Todd children in Peking, June 1934.

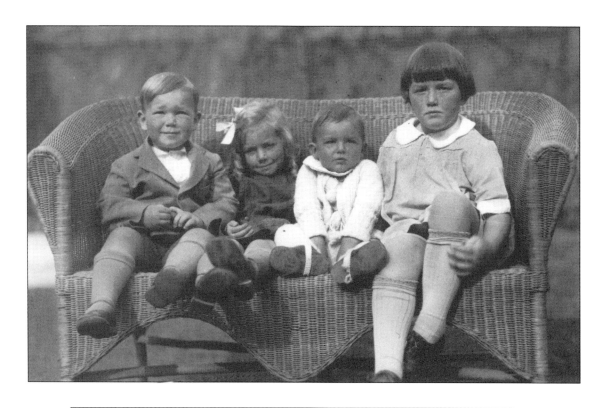

their father's hands while walking up the front of his legs and flipping over back-wards in a somersault). And there were always special outings together when Daddy was home even for only a few days.

LOST DIAMOND

In the summer of 1934 at Pei Tai Ho, one evening at dinner Lois noticed the diamond was missing from her engagement ring. She thought back over the events of the day and wondered where she might have lost her diamond. The day's activities had included playing on the beach, building sand castles, and swimming with the children at Baby Beach in the morning; making her medical rounds on donkey-back through the hills of Pei Tai Ho; playing several sets of tennis on the clay courts; and swimming and playing with the children at Big Beach. She *knew* she would find her lost diamond and organized a search for it the next morning.

Everyone in the American community began sifting the sand on the beaches with sieves; swimming with eyes open under the water looking for her diamond on the ocean floor at the two beaches where she had been swimming; sweeping and sifting the dust on the clay tennis courts; and retracing the trail she rode by donkey over the hills on her medical rounds. The search continued for many days with all ages taking part. After two weeks of searching for the dia-mond without success, many helpers came to the conclusion that the diamond would never be found. Lois never gave up; she was certain she would find it even-tually; and she did.

A few weeks after her diamond was lost, baby Hewlett became sick and developed a high fever. She asked Dr. Armstrong if he would come to the house at East Cliff to see her baby. By the time Dr. Armstrong arrived the baby had finally fallen asleep and Lois did not want him to be awakened by the doctor's loud, booming voice. When she stepped outside the house and off the veranda to ask Dr. Armstrong to keep his voice down so as not to awaken the baby, she saw her diamond sparkle in the crushed seashell path. She walked over to the dia-mond and picked it out of the crushed seashells which were four to six inches deep and were repeatedly churned by the donkey's hooves several times each day. Lois had great faith, determination, patience, and perseverance; she never lost faith, even when others had given up, and the possiblity of finding the diamond seemed remote and improbable.

FAMILY TRAVELS TO AMERICA TO MEET RELATIVES

In April 1935 the Todd family departed by ship from Shanghai on the *President Coolidge* so the four Todd children could meet their relatives in America. Stops in Japan at Kobe and Yokohama were followed by very rough seas until arrival in Honolulu on May 3. It was a rough crossing with Elinor seasick most of the time and the ship arriving in San Francisco on May 8. The family had brief visits with Julian's brother Walter in Oakland and Julian's sister Donna and her husband, John McBryan, while the ship was unloading and loading cargo. Before the ship resumed its journey to Los Angeles with the Todd family aboard, Julian gave his father's gold watch to his son Robert, from his first marriage.

Morris and Gladys Pendleton, Mother Pendleton, and Adaline met the ship when it arrived in San Pedro on May 12. After going through customs, the family spent time in Claremont where the children enjoyed getting acquainted with their Grandmother Pendleton, while Julian kept busy with business appointments in Los Angeles. On May 22 Julian departed by train to Colorado for a visit with his brother, Alfred Todd, who practiced law in Lamar. Julian continued by train via Denver to New York, arriving on June 1 for appointments. June 8 he went to Washington, D.C. to visit his brother Laurence Todd, journalist, and for appointments.

Returning by train via Knoxville and New Orleans to visit engineering friends, he met Lois and the four children in Berkeley to drive north along the California coast to Eugene, Oregon, arriving June 24. After visits with Julian's sister Vera and Mother Todd, Julian returned to Los Angeles by train for another week of appointments. The family stayed in a rented house in Eugene for an extended visit.

Mother Pendleton arrived in Eugene on July 9 to care for the children so Lois, Julian, and his sister Donna could take a month long auto trip to see Bonneville Dam and other reclamation projects and visit several national parks. They stopped at Mount Ranier, Coeur D'Alene, Kootenay, Lake Louise, Banff, Yoho, Waterton Lake, Glacier Park, Yellowstone Park, Grand Teton Park, and the Black Hills. Julian, Lois, and Donna returned to Eugene via Denver, Rocky Mountain National Park, Grand Lake, Salt Lake City, and Twin Falls, Idaho, arriving in Eugene on August 16. Adaline, Lois's sister, helped Mother Pendleton care for the four lively little Todds. The family left on August 28 for California via the Oregon coast, Reedsport and Crescent City.

There were visits to Saratoga and Palo Alto, then Yosemite and Lake Elinor, then south to Sequoia Park, and back to Claremont by September 6. Julian went to San Francisco on September 24 to deliver 114 ancient Chinese bronzes from his collection to the De Young Museum in San Francisco on loan.

Early on September 30 the Todd family arrived in Los Angeles to board the ship, *President Hoover*, for their long journey back home to Peking. The ship

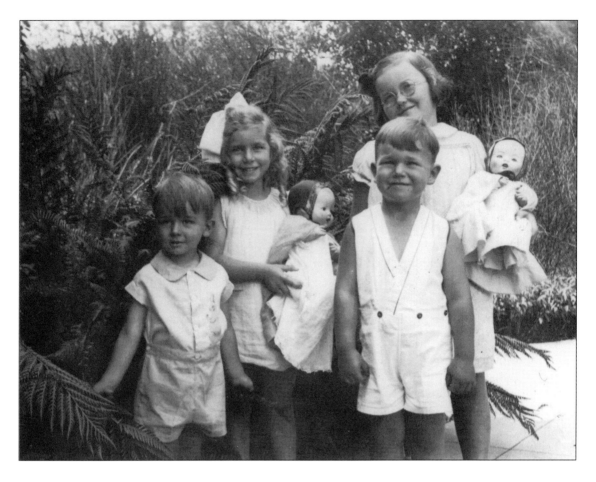

Todd children visiting Grandmother Pendleton in Claremont, California, 1935.

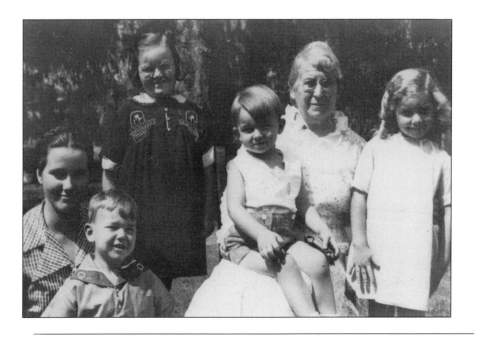

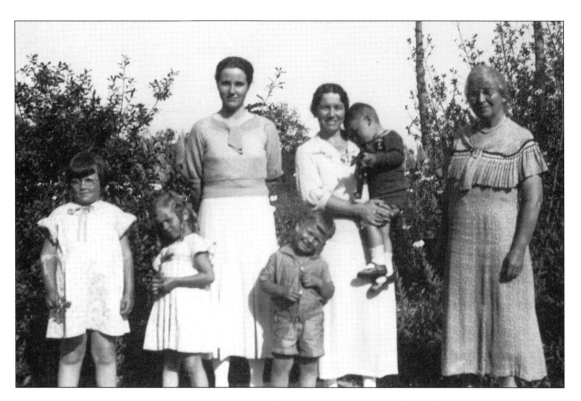

Adaline, Lois, and mother Jessie Pendleton with the four Todd children, 1935.

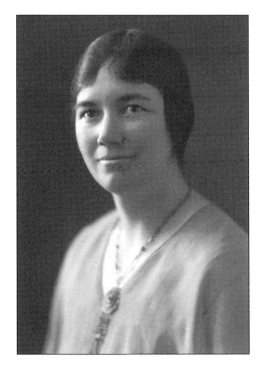

Lois Pendleton Todd, M.D. in 1935.

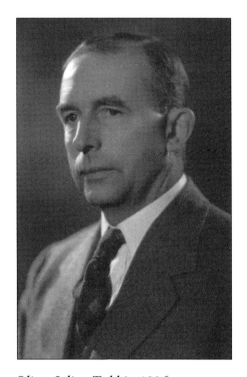

Oliver Julian Todd in 1936.

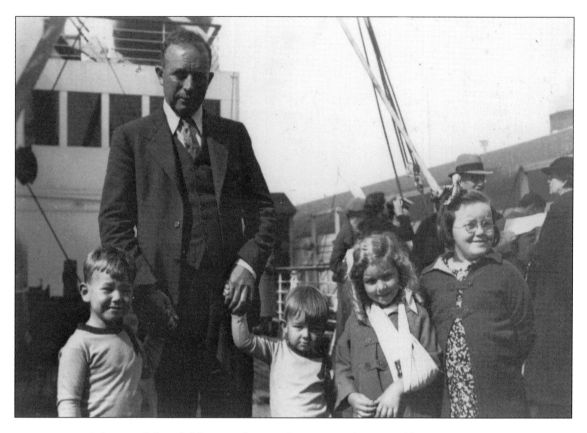

Julian with his children on ship ready to return home to China in 1935. Below: On the sand dunes at Pei Tai Ho, July 1936: Dr. Margaret Tucker (left), Dr. Alma Cooke (medical school classmate of Lois), Hewlett, Dr. Lois Todd, Elinor, Doris, and James.

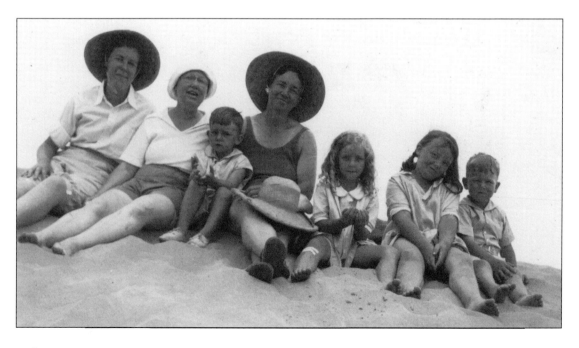

stopped in San Francisco, Honolulu, Kobe and Yokohama, arriving in Shanghai on October 23. The family arrived by train in Peiping (Peking) on October 25, 1935.

The Todd children grew and flourished and Lois kept busy with providing medical care to Americans in Peking and some clinical teaching at P.U.M.C. Julian continued to spend most of his time in his civil engineering field work.

BALLET LESSONS

When Doris and Elinor were six and four and a half years old, respectively, Lois enrolled them in ballet dancing classes in Peking with a British ballet teacher named Miss Billie Thunder. Doris and Elinor attended weekly dance classes, including basic ballet, interpretive dance, and later tap dancing, for the next four years until their departure to America in 1938. Elinor, although shy, was petite and graceful. She, especially, loved the dancing classes and frequently had leading roles in the annual dance recitals, complete with elaborate handmade costumes.

JAPANESE OCCUPATION

The summer of 1937 the train trip to Pei Tai Ho was complicated by Japanese occupation forces seizing the trains for their troop transport, causing other rail cars to be put on sidelines for hours to allow the troop trains through. For the return to Peking later that

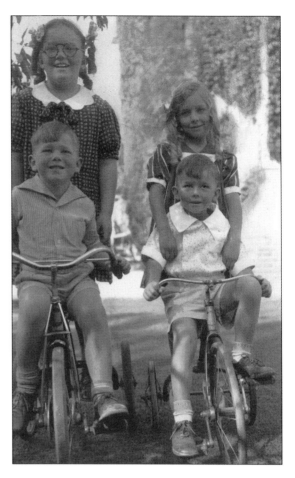

Todd children, Christmas 1936.

Below: Playing wedding at Pei Tai Ho, July 1937: Doris, Hewlett, Elinor, and James.

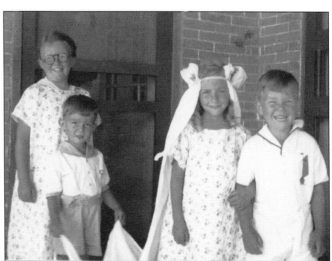

summer Julian arranged for some baggage cars to carry the American families home from Pei Tai Ho. The journey was rough, hot and slow, but all reached home safely.

Peking peacefully surrendered to the Japanese in 1937, opening the city gates and welcoming the Japanese troops rather than risk damage to the many historic treasures in the capitol city: Forbidden City (Imperial Palace), Temple of Heaven, Pei Hai, Summer Palace, and many others.

When Chiang Kai Shek and his generals decided to blow up with dynamite the dikes harnessing the Yellow River, in order to flood the plains in an attempt to stop the Japanese invasion, Lois and Julian realized it was time to leave China and to take their family home to America. Julian knew when his 20 years of engineering work was intentionally destroyed by the Chinese government, he would be unable to continue his work. The time had come to go home to the United States of America. War was imminent.

JOURNEY HOME TO AMERICA

By the spring of 1938, Julian arranged for visas through the American Consul in Peking, Oliver Edmund Clubb. He booked travel home by steamship, the only means available in those days. At 4:00 A.M. on April 22, 1938 the family left their home in Peking, traveling seven hours by train to Tientsin and then by tender into the Yellow Sea where they were transferred to *Choan Maru*, a Japanese officer ship, near Taku at 6:15 P.M. to continue their journey to Kobe, Japan, arriving 8:30 A.M. on April 26, 1938.

The family went by electric train to Kyoto for sightseeeing and to purchase a Satsuma tea set. Other outings during the week included trips to the Kobe Zoo, visiting friends on the faculty at Kobe College, and a trip to Nara to see the deer and temples. On May 1 Julian purchased a beautiful Satsuma bowl and vase for Lois. The next morning the United States Dollar Line's steamship, the *President Taft*, was allowed to come into port to pick up American passengers and their cargo, sailing for America at 6:00 P.M. on May 2, 1938. On May 3 the ship arrived in Yokohama where the Americans were held for medical inspection. Eight hours later the ship was allowed to continue its journey to Hawaii.

Time during the journey by steamship was passed reading, playing deck tennis and shuffleboard, singing, visiting with the other passengers, and movies in the evening. Lois organized school classes for the children when they were not seasick. On May 11 the ship arrived in Honolulu, docking at 11:30 A.M. and sailing again at midnight.

On May 17 the *President Taft* entered the Golden Gate, docking in San Francisco just before noon. It took all afternoon to get through customs with the family's 48 pieces of baggage including trunks and crates of ancient Chinese bronzes, Julian's art collection, and hand-made Chinese rugs from their home in Peking. After two busy days of visiting relatives and shopping, the family took the Daylight Limited train to Los Angeles on May 19 to visit Morris and Gladys Pendleton in San Marino and Adaline and Mother Pendleton in Claremont. On May 25 Lois and Julian spent the entire day at Wilmington getting their freight through customs.

On May 27 Julian took the coach train east to Phoenix, Tucson, Albuquerque, and La Junta, Colorado, where his brother Alfred met him and took him by car to his home in Lamar for a two day visit, then on to Kansas City, Des Moines, Chicago, and Ann Arbor, Michigan, for two days. On June 2 he traveled by train to New York, where he spent the next two weeks on business calls and on errands. On June 17 Julian was back in Ann Arbor to visit his alma mater, University of Michigan. He visited relatives in Kalamazoo then returned to Ann Arbor to see the Hydraulic Laboratory at the University. He called on the Dean of the Engineering Department to leave a copy of his book *Two Decades in China* and he spoke to the Chinese students studying engineering at the University.

While Julian traveled, Lois and their children relaxed in Claremont at her mother's home and at her brother Morris's beach house on Balboa Island. When Julian returned from the east, he spent time at Balboa Island working on his article on the Yellow River work. Lois and Julian celebrated their wedding anniversary on July 2 at Balboa Island with a motor launch trip in the afternoon and a beach party.

With the help of Morris Pendleton, Lois and Julian bought a 1938 Packard car in Los Angeles for $925 plus 3% sales tax. On July 4 the family of seven, including four children plus Adaline, left Claremont in the 1938 Packard to drive 465 miles to Oakland, with Lois and Adaline taking turns driving. On July 6 Lois and Julian drove to Palo Alto to look at houses to buy or rent, as Lois had obtained a position as student health physician at Stanford.

CHAPTER 7

Palo Alto: Balancing Career and Family

The journey home from China was over and Doctor Lois and her family were ready to begin a new chapter in their lives in 1938. They established their new home in California, about thirty miles north of her childhood home in Saratoga. Lois and Julian selected Palo Alto for a home because Lois had obtained a position on the Stanford University faculty as student health physician, working with Helen Brenton Pryor, M.D., providing medical care to women students enrolled at Stanford. Dr. Helen Pryor had been a student at University of California School of Medicine, a year or two behind Lois.

On July 6 Lois and Julian motored through the Stanford campus, looked at three homes in Palo Alto, and visited several friends in the vicinity. The next morning, with their four children ranging from ages ten to five years and Lois's sister, Adaline, in their 1938 Packard, they drove north along the California coast to Reedsport, Oregon, then inland to Eugene for a family vacation.

Julian's sister Vera and her husband Ralph Crow lived in a pleasant home on Willamette Avenue on the outskirts of Eugene. Their home was surrounded by a spacious garden and fruit orchard. Next door lived Vera and Julian's mother, Julia Farrand Todd. The alert 91 year old Todd family matriarch occupied her own home, assisted by a housekeeper. Mother Todd's little home was surrounded by a modest orchard of hazelnut, or filbert trees.

Vera had prepared the Crow house (her husband's childhood home) for housing Adaline, Lois, Julian, and their four lively youngsters. The old Crow house was across open fields toward Spencer's Butte from Vera and Ralph's home and had extensive wild blackberry patches around it and across the road. The next four days Lois and Julian spent on errands, visiting, getting their auto repaired, and making preparations for climbing Mount Hood with purchases of supplies, climbing rope, and hiking boots. Julian also edited his irrigation paper for the Civil Engineering Journal and had Adaline retype it, mailing it back to New York to meet a publishing deadline.

On July 12 Vera and Ralph agreed to take care of the children. The next morning Adaline, Lois, and Julian left at 6:00 A.M. via Multnomah Falls and Hood River to Timberline Lodge on the south flank of Mount Hood. On July 14 at 4:15 A.M., Adaline, Lois, and Julian began their climb of Mount Hood, arriving at the top at 11:20 A.M. The last part of the hike was slow due to soft, melting snow. They followed a group of C.C.C. men and their supervisor, using 600 feet of rope up the last steep climb. Staying an hour and a half on top, they ate their lunch and were back to camp by 3:30 P.M., returning to Portland for the night.

Their four children, Doris, Elinor, James, and Hewlett, enjoyed leisurely days hunting for wild strawberries on the hill, picking wild blackberries across the road, and standing on a straight back chair cranking the old Victrola in the Crow house to play tubular records such as "Daisie, Daisie, Give Me Your Answer True," "T'was Only a Pansy Blossom," and "Red River Valley." They also enjoyed visiting Grandmother Todd (who was born in 1847), hearing the wonderful stories about her youth and how she witnessed President Abraham Lincoln giving a campaign speech from the rear of a train in Indiana when he was running for re-election and she was a young schoolteacher.

On July 18 Julian went on the Southern Pacific train to Salt Lake City to an engineering convention where he had been invited to give a speech on his engineering work in China. At this convention he met several of his engineering classmates from University of Michigan engineering class of 1908.

By July 23 he was back in Eugene preparing to take an auto tour with his older brother, Victor, to engineering projects Victor had worked on in Washington state. Enroute to Seattle on July 25 Lois and Julian arrived at Paradise Valley on the slope of Mount Ranier. Julian intended to climb the mountain, but the guides and rangers discouraged it because of a large crevasse. So they hiked only to Glacier Vista and back. That evening he found a man who was willing to climb with him the next morning to Muir Cabin halfway up the mountain. At 5:10 A.M. the next morning they were hiking to Muir Cabin. The next few days

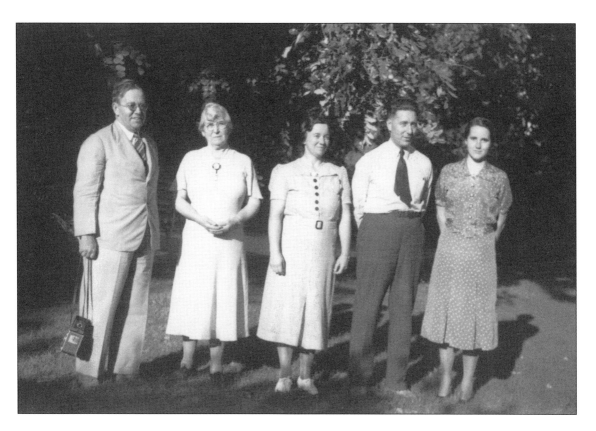

Pendleton family reunion in Palo Alto at "Seven Pines":
Robert, mother Jessie, Lois, Morris, and Adaline.

were spent touring Diablo Dam and Grand Coulee Dam. Adaline was taking care of the children in Eugene during this week.

Vera and Lois went to a women's camp at Florence, a seashore community west of Eugene. Three days later Adaline, Julian, and the children drove to the coast to pick up Vera and Lois at Florence, where the children frolicked on the beach, enjoyed a picnic lunch, and waded in the tide pools near the Seal Caves.

The family drove southeast to Crater Lake to view and wonder at that beautiful, deep blue body of water, then drove southwest to Crescent City, continuing the journey south along the California coast the next day to Walter and Ida Todd's home in Oakland.

Lois and Julian spent more time looking for a house in Palo Alto and helping Adaline to find housing in San Francisco for her clinical years at University of California School of Medicine. The next day Lois, Julian, the four children and Adaline drove to Claremont, enjoying a lunch stop at the Big Sur redwoods and arriving in Claremont by midnight at Mother Pendleton's home.

The family enjoyed a few days at the beach where Morris and Gladys Pendleton hosted a big dinner party at their beach house on Balboa Island for seventeen family members.

On August 17 Lois and Julian went early by car to Wilmington to arrange for shipping their freight north to San Francisco. After five more days of business appointments, errands and social calls, the family left Claremont by car at 6:00 A.M. on August 22 for Oakland. Lois and Julian spent all the next day in Palo Alto looking for a house. By 7:00 P.M., they had signed a contract to rent a small furnished house along San Francisquito Creek, within walking distance of Lytton Elementary School.

By 8:40 P.M. that evening Julian was on the coach train south to Los Angeles where he had been invited to be one of three speakers at the Authors Club the next day. He took the evening coach train north after giving the speech and was back in Palo Alto at 6:52 A.M. the next morning.

Lois and Julian went over the new house to estimate storage space, bought a desk, dishes, and sewing machine, and then went to San Francisco to see about their freight shipped from Los Angeles.

On August 27 the family left Walter and Ida's home in Oakland and moved to Grant and Clotilde Taylor's place in Redwood City for five days, in quarters over their garage, while waiting for their freight to arrive from Los Angeles. Lois and the children and Clotilde went horse-back riding in the mornings and played with the Taylor family menagerie in the afternoons. The Taylors had four children, about ten years older than the Todd children, and many pets. The cats and dogs were all trained to do amazing tricks such as going down slides, swinging, jumping through hoops, and ringing a call bell when they wanted to ride in their own pet elevator, a wooden box on rope with pulley, to an upstairs window.

The Todd family took auto trips to Crystal Springs Lake and along Skyline Boulevard to the Pendleton family's mountain place, Minnewawa, in the Santa Cruz mountains above Saratoga to pick apples and pears in the family orchard.

On September 1 the family moved to their newly rented home at 750 Palo Alto Avenue in Palo Alto. The freight arrived at 11:00 A.M. and was unloaded by 1:00 P.M.; the men worked for two hours carrying trunks to the basement and rearranging boxes in the garage. The children's bicycle, tricycle, wagon, and scooters arrived before noon to their delight. The next week was spent opening boxes and crates, unpacking books, and getting the family organized.

By September 8 Julian was making contacts to sell some of his ancient Chinese bronze mirrors, writing a story for the "Saturday Evening Post," and

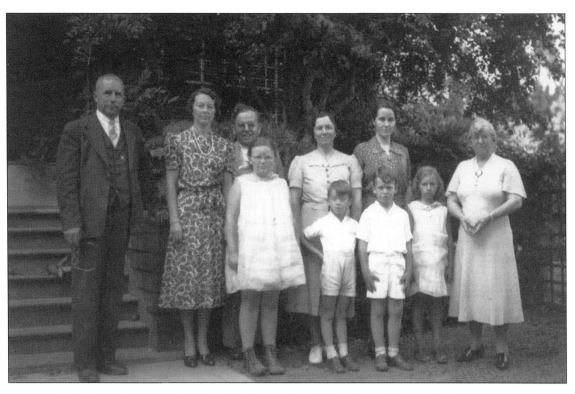

Family gathering at "Seven Pines": Adults left to right: Julian Todd, Gladys Pendleton (wife of Morris), Robert Pendleton, Lois Todd, Adaline and Jessie Pendleton. Children left to right: Doris, Hewlett, James, and Elinor.

packing for a trip to Hetch Hetchy Dam in the Sierra Nevada mountains. At 5:30 A.M. the next morning, Julian, his brother Walter, and an engineering friend were on their way by car to Hetch Hetchy, near Yosemite, where Julian had worked as a young engineer before World War I. He had camped for a year at Lake Elinor near Tuolumne Meadows and had done the initial surveys for the city of San Francisco for the construction of Hetch Hetchy Dam, which became the source of San Francisco's water supply. After spending the night in a cabin at South Fork they hiked to Lake Elinor (for which his second daughter was named) early the next morning and Julian took photos of the place he had lived and worked thirty years earlier and of Hetchy Hetchy Dam, built during his China years. (The spelling of Lake Elinor, the British spelling, has been changed to Eleanor, the French spelling, on more recent California maps.)

September 11 was a busy day spent opening boxes, washing walls, and entertaining family and friends. Walter and Ida Todd and their ten year old son Ted came for lunch; Joe Kahn and his wife Mabel and grandchild, Robert Todd (Julian's son by his first marriage), came for dinner. On September 12 the four children started school and the busy routine of the household became established.

Lois participated in the PTA activities of each school where her children were enrolled. One year they were in four different schools, meaning four different PTA's in which Lois participated.

The Todd children spoke Chinese to each other in their play at home, as it is a simpler language gramatically. However, when their new friends overheard the Chinese spoken and began to refer to the children as "foreigners," Doris, Elinor, James, and Hewlett promptly dropped their Chinese and refused to speak it with their parents at the dinner table. They did not want to be considered different or foreigners by their new American friends.

Julian made, on the average, two trips a week by train to San Franciso for luncheon meetings and professional contacts, and spent increasing time on preparing manuscripts for publication. Lois began her job as physician at the Women's Health Service at Stanford University on September 25, 1938. She had to find baby sitters for the children as Julian was out and about with his many activities and rarely at home. He was much too engrossed in his projects to keep an eye on the children. Lois soon hired Pearl to be live-in housekeeper, to cook, and to help with the children.

Julian had served in the Army Corps of Engineers in World War I in France, being discharged with the rank of Major. In 1938, with the war accelerating in China, he decided to apply for reinstatement in Army Officers Reserve. He also applied to the Federal Power Commission and the Bureau of Reclamation for a job. He applied to the State Civil Engineering License Board and received his license to practice engineering in California. But finding an engineering job at age fifty-eight, after being out of the country for eighteen years, proved to be a prolonged and frustrating search.

Lois and Julian continued to look at houses for sale, and on October 16 bought a small house in Menlo Park only for investment purposes. Julian named this property "Mr. MacGregor's Garden" after the story of Peter Cottontail. There were guava, lemon, olive, almond, and walnut trees, and lots of old tools in the tool shed and in the basement. A renter was found for this property. Lois and Julian continued their search for another larger house to buy, as it was obvious that the family was bursting at the seams in the little house where they were living on Palo Alto Avenue.

HOME

Eventually they found a wonderful, big old house on spacious grounds at 1445 Hamilton Avenue in the Crescent Park area of Palo Alto. It had originally been the private home of a physician who had it custom built in 1906 on the outskirts, east of town; later it became a boarding school. The present owners had raised their four children in the house and modernized the house in 1930. On November 5, 1938, Lois and Julian signed the papers to purchase Seven Pines from the Deering family.

Home at last, and what a wonderful home it was, nestled in a garden paradise. The entire two-thirds of an acre included seven magnificent Monterey pine trees reaching 50 to 60 feet into the air. It was beautifully landscaped. There were three handsome southern magnolia trees in the front yard that perfumed the air every May through July with their large creamy white, fragrant blossoms the size of dinner plates. A Chinese wisteria vine was festooned over the front porch and entry with its lavendar blooms in grape-like clusters delightfully scenting the air every April. A young Ginkgo tree from China was planted in the front lawn and turned a glorious gold every autumn before shedding its leaves for the winter. Several English holly bushes, both male and female, which became small trees, sparkling with shiny red berries in the winter months, surrounded the front lawn. There were Toyon (California holly) bushes, ceanothus (wild lilac), and pittusporum, as well as two varieties of flowering plum trees in the front yard, also loquat trees, and a large, gnarled carob tree near the front porch. Paths paved with pine needles and edged with pine logs wound through the front garden, between the front lawn and the street, fondly referred to as "the jungle" by the Todd children—a wonderful place to play hide-and-seek.

Between the front yard and the back yard, on the north side of the house, was a formal rose garden which became the pride and joy of Doctor Lois. In the evenings, after work and after feeding the family, she would work in her rose garden, pruning, watering, and fertilizing her roses. There were three rectangular plots 16 by 28 feet, each surrounded by a pruned box-wood hedge about 15 inches high, with 20 or so prize hybrid rose bushes in each plot. There were also two rose arbors connecting the plots at the north end of the rose garden, one with Hoover roses and the other with Talisman roses. She delighted in taking fresh roses from her garden to her office and to her friends several times a week.

Another special hobby of hers was raising tuberous begonias, large and spectacular blooms that look like camellias, roses, peonies, or carnations with colors varying from white, yellow, orange, or red to pink, peach, and apricot. She purchased the special tubers from a hybrid grower in Capitola and lovingly raised them in the front yard under the shade of the large Monterey pines. She would be up early in the mornings to water her begonias before going to work and would water them again in the evening if the day had been hot.

The back yard included a wood-yard surrounded by wild cherry trees, where branches and logs from tree trimming were stored and compost pits contained leaves and grass clippings for making mulch for the garden. Also in the back yard were American holly, loquat trees, bay laurel trees, a huge Monterey pine, a lawn surrounded by perennials, acanthus, agapanthus (Lily of the Nile), cotoneaster, and acacia trees, and a two car garage and driveway turn-around.

The children had two primary responsibilities in the extensive gardens at Seven Pines: mowing the front and back lawns every week with an old-fashioned reel hand-push mower and gathering snails by the bucketful from the rose garden, acanthus, and begonias. Doris mowed the lawns until Elinor was big enough to take over the job, which paid 35 cents total. When James and Hewlett reached age ten or twelve they mowed the lawns. Julian, when he was at home, diligently swept the driveway (all 200 plus feet of it) each morning and raked leaves and pine needles from the front and back lawns daily.

A hedge of Mermaid roses and a row of Red Hot Pokers ran along the front fence adjacent to the sidewalk. Trimming the rose hedge regularly to keep pedestrians from being injured by the rose thorns while walking by was a difficult and "thorny" job. The walnut trees in front and in the back yard bore nuts every fall which the children harvested by knocking them down with bamboo poles, then scrambling on the ground in the ivy to gather them up. These were spread on boards in the back yard to dry, then hulled by gloved hands because of the indelible stain, then dried some more, bagged, and stored in the basement for use in baking and cooking.

The house was spacious with a screened porch across the front of the house, a large library/living room, and dining room, separated by a large foyer and stairway, all trimmed with fir woodwork in dark walnut stain, and pairs of large sliding pocket doors that could separate the main rooms from the foyer; a walk-in pantry, kitchen, laundry room, bathroom, and maid's room completed the main floor. A large stairway and banister led from the foyer to a landing and then split with one flight of stairs continuing ahead to a large glassed and screened bedroom plus bath (above the laundry room, bathroom, and maid's room on the main floor) and the main stair continuing to the right to the upstairs foyer which was surrounded by four more bedrooms and a bathroom.

Three of these bedrooms were large with a walk-in closet connecting two of them. One of these large bedrooms facing the front of the house, the master bedroom, had an attached glassed and screened porch which served as a nursery when Hewlett was little and later as a sewing room. The view of the front garden from this sewing room was choice. The air wafting in these windows was fragrant from the magnolia tree just to the west and from the wisteria and rose garden below and was filled with the serenade of bird songs. Lois and her daughters enjoyed reading and sewing in this delightful room. Doris and Elinor made most of their own clothes beginning at age ten to twelve on an old White treadle sewing machine. Lois made sleeping bags for her children to take to summer camp as the family budget was too tight to purchase sleeping bags. Lois even wrote to her brother Morris in Los Angeles to ask him to obtain the extra long industrial grade zippers to go around three sides of each sleeping bag, as these zippers were not available in the stores in Palo Alto.

The other large bedroom on the front of the house became Julian's study, filled with his books, files, photos, and mementos. This room on the southwest corner was sunny, bright, and pleasant, a spacious area for him to work on his correspondence and extensive writing of manuscripts and articles, keeping his account ledgers, and handling his professional and household business.

PROJECTS

Soon after moving into their new home, Julian decided to undertake a major engineering feat with the help of three men and his four small children. He planned to excavate a basement under the entire house, where there was only a concrete pad just large enough for the furnace and water heater. He wanted a full concrete basement for more storage space for trunks, crates, books, home-canned foods, and suitcases, and room for a ping-pong table.

In January 1939 three men helped Julian excavate the basement with hand shovels and filled buckets which the children carried up the stairs and emptied in the back yard, creating a hill. The project continued daily until the excavation was completed a week later. Next Julian framed the ledges, vertical walls, and floor during the next two days in preparation for pouring the concrete. The hired men helped him pour concrete thc next three days, and another day was required to finish the concrete. The project was completed in two weeks and was a great success.

A deep hole suddenly appeared in the back lawn one day a few years later, when the wooden planks over an old cistern rotted and gave way, and a section of the back lawn collapsed into the deep, dangerous cistern. The children were again enlisted and the dirt in the hill created from the basement excavation was shoveled again and carried by the bucketful to fill the cistern under the back lawn.

In September 1945 Julian decided to pave the long gravel driveway and turn-around in concrete using his own children for labor. The basement construction was such a successful project that he decided to make a concrete driveway. This project was an easier one as no excavation was involved. With the help of James and Hewlett, he built the wooden frames along the two outer edges of the driveway, nearly 200 feet from the garage to the street, plus the arcing turnaround past the back door of the house toward the wood yard. When the concrete was delivered, all four children spread the concrete between the frames with rakes and hoes, then smoothed it until even. The project took several days to complete. Doris, Elinor, James, and Hewlett were older at the time of this project and had another experience in hard manual labor (coolie labor). They considered their father a harsh and demanding task master. O. J. Todd, the engineer and efficiency expert, barked orders at his children while working side by side with them, admonishing them to work harder and to work faster. He taught them the work ethic and the valuable lessons of self-sufficiency, perseverance, tenacity, and the satisfaction of success in completing a project, from planning to execution. These were important lessons for life.

RECREATION

During 1939 the World's Fair was held in San Francisco Bay on Treasure Island, a man-made extension of Yerba Buena Island. The fair was named Golden Gate Exposition. Lois and Julian and their four children made seven trips during the year to see the various exhibits in the educational and mind-expanding World's Fair. The entire family enjoyed these all day expeditions to the Golden Gate Exposition. During their final visit to the World's Fair they adopted two free kittens, carrying them to the car in empty popcorn bags, much to the children's delight.

Other family outings included the De Young Museum, Japanese Tea Garden, and Fleishacker Zoo in Golden Gate Park, and the Museum of Natural History in San Francisco. Several auto trips each year took the family to their mountain place, Minnewawa, above Saratoga. There the family enjoyed hiking, climbing the ladders at Castle Rock to explore its caves, and picking pears and apples in their mountain orchard.

The summer of 1939, and many summers thereafter, Doris and Elinor took swimming lessons and other classes at Stanford. All four children enrolled in a variety of classes at the Palo Alto Community Center each summer including theater, science, ceramics, tennis, and Christmas pageant, transporting themselves by bicycle. As the children increased their tennis skills they began to play tennis with their parents, in addition to entering singles and doubles tennis tournaments at the Palo Alto Community Center.

The Todd children rode their bicycles everywhere, including riding their bikes to school every day. As the children outgrew a bicycle it was passed along to a younger sibling, and another used bicycle was purchased by the one needing a larger bike.

There were family outings to pick raspberries, cherries, plums, apricots, peaches, pears, and apples in the various fruit orchards in Santa Clara valley that advertised "Pick your own fruit." These outings were followed by home canning and making jams, jellies, and fruit juices for homemade punch.

In June 1939 the family visited Robert Todd, Julian's son by his first wife Rheta; he was working at a gas station and was a college student at the College of Pacific in Stockton.

LONG ABSENCES

Late in June 1940, O. J. Todd received a job appointment from the Denver office of the Bureau of Reclamation, doing field study of water diversion projects in New Mexico and Arizona. After a big family reunion at Seven Pines on July 4th, Julian left by train on July 7 for Denver. The Shirley Savoy Hotel in downtown Denver became his home when he was working in the Denver office. July 15 he drove 486 miles to Albuqueque where he had an office for his field work studying the middle fork of the Rio Grande, water diversion projects, and silt studies in New Mexico. He also worked out of the Conservancy office in Socorro, New Mexico.

Julian was gone for the next two and a half years, except for each Christmas when he came home by train to spend a week with his family in Palo Alto. Lois traveled by train from San Francisco to Denver to visit Julian each summer for a week to celebrate their wedding anniversary together.

STANFORD

Doctor Lois enjoyed her work at Stanford from the beginning. She and her friend Dr. Helen Pryor worked well together and had a very helpful and supportive staff of nurses to assist them in providing high quality medical care to the women students enrolled at Stanford University. Their offices were conveniently located in the Women's Gym, across the street from the women's dormitories. The male physicians had separate offices in the Men's Gym, near the men's dormitories, providing medical care to the male students and varsity athletes.

Work began with a bang at the beginning of each academic year. All new students were required to have a complete physical exam at the Student Health Service, review their medical history with a staff physician, and receive any immunizations needed during their new student orientation. Each morning before clinic hours (8:00 A.M. to 5:00 P.M.) Dr. Lois Todd or Dr. Helen Pryor made rounds on any patients in the infirmary, known as the Rest Home. It was an old family residence, only a short distance from the heart of the Stanford campus, which had been converted to a twelve bed facility for students needing rest, isolation, or nursing care but not requiring acute hospital care. Lois would stop again at the Rest Home on her way home if she had concerns about any patients.

Dr. Lois Todd was given a faculty appointment, Assistant Professor, and taught a class in Hygiene (personal health and preventive medicine). She continued to work full-time at the Student Health Service and to keep her faculty appointment until mandatory retirement at age 65 in 1960. After 22 years of service to Stanford University students, she became emeritus faculty.

Many changes occurred in the Student Health Service over the years. In 1942 due to World War II most of the male physicians were sent to war; so the Men's and Women's Student Health Services were combined at the Women's Gym where Dr. Helen Pryor and Dr. Lois Todd cared for both male and female students. Clinic space was increased by remodeling classroom space at the Women's Gymnasium.

After World War II, Stanford University and Palo Alto Clinic entered into a contract to provide additional physicians and also specialty consultants to augment the physicians on campus. George Houck, M.D., was hired to be medical director of the newly expanded and enlarged Stanford University Health Service at the end of World War II. Dr. Lois Todd worked under Dr. Houck until her retirement in 1960. She was the only full-time woman physician on the staff of the Stanford Health Service during these years.

Doctor Lois was active in the Faculty Women's Club during her 22 years at Stanford. She participated actively in many campus activities and enjoyed including her children in attending the Stanford Chapel on Sunday to hear sermons by renowned preachers such as Dr. Elton Trueblood (Stanford chaplain), Reinhold Niebuhr, Howard Thurman and others. She bought season tickets to the concert series each year, taking her children to chamber music and symphony concerts. She loved classical music. The Tuesday evening series of weekly travelogues and lectures was another favorite family activity through the school year.

During the summer session she enrolled her children in special enrichment programs for children of Stanford faculty such as puppet workshops, reading workshops, and writing workshops. Lois's career at Stanford continued to be a source of much challenge, stimulation, and satisfaction over the years. And it kept the roof over the family's head, as Julian had difficulty finding regular work because of his age and his many years abroad.

Dr. Lois Todd was beloved by the Stanford students. When son James lived and worked in New England he met many Stanford alumni who remembered with fondness Dr. Lois Todd, and how much help she was as friend as well as physician. She had several students who were second generation patients -- they sought her out when they became students at Stanford because their parents had been patients of hers while studying at Stanford and recommended her so highly. She was a good listener, a very astute diagnostician and clinician, a caring physician, and a wise counselor. During her Stanford years two of her clinical papers were published in medical journals—one titled "Cat Scratch Fever" and another "Anaphylaxis from Oral Penicillin."

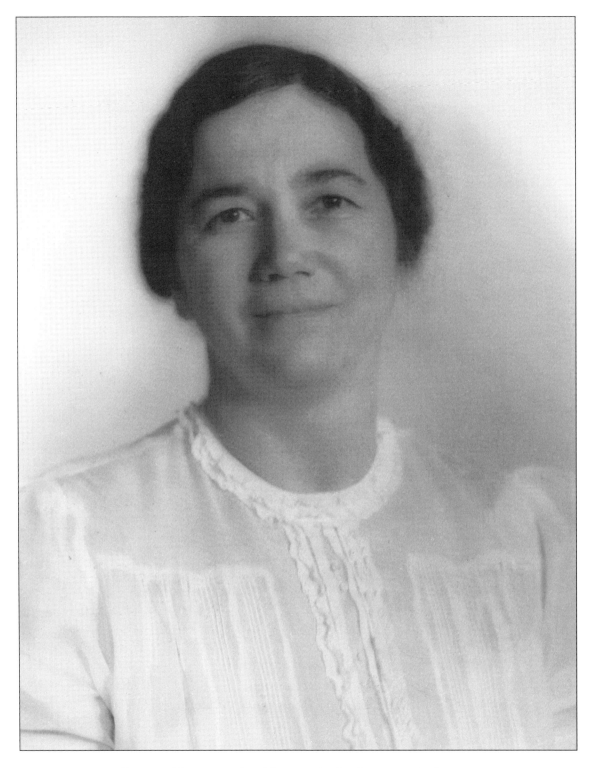

Lois Pendleton Todd, M.D. in her fifties on the faculty at Stanford University.

WORLD WAR II

In January 1943 Julian was hired by the Army Engineers through their Phoenix office and given an urgent project to accomplish from an office in Fort Huachuca. He was assigned to build a prisoner of war camp near Douglas, Arizona along the Mexican border, for German war prisoners. This 2,000 man project was completed in March 1943; papers and equipment were packed and shipped back to Army Engineers headquarters.

Fort Huachuca and Douglas were in rattlesnake country. O. J. Todd learned to catch them and kill them. He collected the rattles from the rattlesnakes in a cigar box and brought them home to his children as souvenirs.

On March 16, 1943 Julian noticed vision loss following a one car accident in which he lost control of the car on a gravel road with a soft shoulder; the car jumped a pasture fence and landed in a field with a jolt. When he returned home by train from Denver several days later, Lois took him to Stanford Hospital in San Francisco where a detached retina was diagnosed. Eye surgery with platinum pins to hold the retina to the back of the orbit was performed on March 27. He was immobilized in bed with bandages over both eyes and sandbags on each side of his head to hold his head still while his retina healed. This was difficult for such an active, vigorous man. Two weeks later the bandages were removed and pin-hole papers were placed over both eyes to prevent movement of his eyes. He was released from the hospital to continue his convalescence at home. On May 18 the pin-hole papers were removed and he was able to write again; 60% per cent of his vision had been restored.

In June 1943 he was hired by U. S. Engineers, Los Angeles office, to work on the Whitewater flood project and the La Quinta flood project. Lois visited him in Los Angeles for four days in July to celebrate their anniversary and also visited her Pendleton relatives in San Marino and Claremont. In August and September he worked on the San Bernardino and Santa Ana flood channel study, including silt research. Lois was with Julian in Los Angeles again in October when he was hospitalized at Cedars of Lebanon for prostate surgery. When he was released from the hospital he convalesced for a week in the San Marino home of Lois's brother Morris and family.

December 24 he took the overnight train from Los Angeles to Palo Alto for Christmas with his family, returning to Los Angeles by train two days later. In January, February, and March he worked on the Los Angeles River Project and the Santa Ynez flood problem. In April he enjoyed ten days of vacation at home in Palo Alto, traveling again by overnight train. He worked with his children in their Victory garden, went with the family to their mountain place, and heard Elinor and Doris sing in the church choir. By mid-April he was back at the Los Angeles office.

An airmail letter arrived on June 10 from Lowdermilk, longtime engineering friend, saying, "O. J. Todd will be needed in China". Julian was intrigued and excited at the prospect, but continued his work in Los Angeles on the Santa Clara River flood studies from June through October 1944. Lois visited him for a week in July to celebrate their wedding anniversary.

Naval Intelligence Office in San Francisco requested Julian to report to their office the end of October for two weeks of meetings in which they requested him to share his information, maps, and photos of China with them. On weekends Lois and Julian played tennis with their children. In mid-November he had returned to Los Angeles for a week of work, then returned home again by train for another two weeks of sharing his China material with Army Intelligence in San Francisco, particularly regarding his wide knowledge of Shansi province.

November 26 he applied for employment with United Nations Relief and Rehabilitaion Agency (UNRRA). He returned to his work in Los Angeles by train for two more weeks of work. He was home again to Palo Alto for Christmas and enjoyed a week with his family, playing tennis with Elinor and the boys. In January 1945 Col. Thompson predicted O. J. Todd would be called to China for service within six months.

In February Julian began Chinese language studies while working in Los Angeles on the San Diego tidal basin problem. On March 24 he returned home to Palo Alto for Easter and received a letter from Lois's cousin Phil Lawton that he had read a news item in the Stockton newspaper stating that Robert Todd (Julian's son by his first marriage) had been killed in an airplane accident in Army pilot training in Alabama, survived by his widow the former Jean Taylor of Lodi and their infant daughter, Roberta. Julian was heartbroken as he was very fond of his grown son Robert (named for the Scottish poet Robert Burns). Julian attended Robert's funeral in Stockton on March 27, 1945, and offered financial assistance to his young widow, Jean.

During the following days Doris, Elinor, James, and Hewlett helped their father paint the family house in Palo Alto before he returned to his work in Los Angeles after Easter. In mid-May Julian returned by train to Palo Alto for a final week of meetings with U.S. Army Intelligence in San Francisco and to pick up the pictures, records, and maps that he had loaned to them.

In mid-June 1945 Julian was transferred at his request to the U.S. Engineers office in Sacramento, which was closer to home. During June, July, and August he worked on the Sacramento River tributary studies.

On September 3 he received a letter from UNRRA regarding work. Four days later Hugh Calkins phoned him from Washington, D.C. saying, "UNRRA wants O. J. Todd for China work." On October 15, 1945, the Washington, D.C., UNRRA office teletyped instructions for O. J. Todd to go there for 30 days on detached duty starting at once. At the end of the war in 1945, Julian was hired by UNRRA to return to China to harness the Yellow River, "China's Sorrow", and to return it to the course he had built for it earlier in his career (1920 to 1938).

It was an easier task this time as he had adequate funds and equipment for the job. However, there was a civil war going on between the Nationalists and the Communists who were fighting for control of the country. So this time his task was complicated by having to relocate villages and negotiate with leaders of both the Nationalist and Communist parties involved in the civil war. He hired local laborers and paid them with bags of grain (wheat and millet) as he had done twenty years earlier. But this time he had some sophisticated equipment such as mechanized pile drivers (for setting posts or "piles" the size of telephone poles) to help expedite the work.

After a brief but intense experience of running for Congress in the Democratic primaries for U.S. House of Representatives, following completion of the project of harnessing the Yellow River, O.J. Todd was sent by UNRRA to develop and improve the irrigation system on Taiwan. An urgent need to increase the food production had arisen on this island, the new home for Nationalists who were fleeing mainland China due to the Communist take-over.

During the years of World War II, when Doris and Elinor were in junior high and senior high school, the youngsters were busy during the summer months raising Victory Garden vegetables on the vacant lot next door to their home; this was a fairly common practice during World War II because of the food shortage. Each of the four children planted his or her own plot, selecting seeds, spading the heavy soil, planting, weeding, watering, and harvesting. They competed, marketing their produce to their mother, who paid comparable grocery store prices for the garden-fresh produce. The children raised radishes, onions, carrots, beets, Swiss chard, spinach, several varieties of squash, rhubarb, green beans, tomatoes, lettuce, and artichokes. Each child kept his or her own account ledger for their Victory Garden enterprise, which their father would review when he returned home for a visit. Through the Victory Gardens the children learned the meaning of manual labor, learned about patience and perseverence, experienced competition, and had their first introduction to accounting.

The family also raised chickens and rabbits in their back yard during the war years. There was a war-time lifting of restrictive covenants because of meat rationing and shortage. The children had many daily chores including feeding and watering the chickens, gathering the eggs, and feeding and watering the rabbits. James learned to help his mother butcher the rabbits and chickens to be cooked for the family table. James dried the rabbit pelts and sold them to earn money for his savings account.

Lois bought a cute pair of fluffy baby ducklings one Easter as pets for her children. She selected white Muscovy ducks which are widely used domestically and are quackless, and therefore would not disturb the neighbors. Lois reasoned that the ducks would eat the snails in the garden, reducing plant damage. The children had lost interest in gathering snails for ten cents a bucketful. However "Ping" and "Pong" had no interest in hunting for snails; they had become pets. They perched on the back porch most of the day leaving their droppings on the doorstep, making an unbelievably slippery mess that smelled like a barnyard. The ducks ate snails only when they were fed to them by hand.

Lois became exasperated within a year and decided to have duck dinner. She butchered one of the ducks and roasted it for dinner, but none of the children could eat a bite. "Ping" had been their pet. So during a family conference at dinner that evening, it was decided to release "Pong" at the Yacht Basin to intermingle with the wild ducks. The children checked several times on her well-being and were pleased to see that she was thriving. After some time, partly white ducks appeared among the wild mallard ducks.

During the war years when gasoline was rationed, the family took no vacations, but the children each went to Scout camp every summer. Doris and Elinor went to Sky Meadow, the Girl Scout camp in Big Basin Redwood State Park on the west side of the Santa Cruz mountains, for two weeks each summer starting at age ten. James and Hewlett went to Oljato, the Boy Scout camp at Huntington Lake near Kings Canyon in the Sierras, for two weeks to a month each summer during their scouting years. James became an Eagle Scout and was a camp counselor several summers.

Even though gasoline was rationed, the family saved their ration stamps and had a weekend outing two or three times a year by auto the 50 miles to Minnewawa. A primitive cabin, water pumped from a spring to a water tank on the hill, fruit orchards, and the beautiful redwood gulch for hiking made it an enjoyable and easily accessible outing during those years of gasoline rationing.

Since the cabin had no stove or electricity, Lois would prepare baked beans and Boston brown bread in the fireless cooker (an insulated chest with oven-heated stones placed above and below the kettles of food) so the family could have a hot cooked meal at the end of the day.

PARENTING

Doctor Lois continued her busy dual careers as physician and parent of four lively, precocious adolescents. Julian's long absences due to his work must have been difficult, but she never complained and did a wonderful job of being both father and mother to her children, guiding her flock with considerable wisdom and success. The Palo Alto Times named her 1954 Mother of the Year. (See Family Foundations IV.)

Morris Pendleton, Lois's younger brother, frequently stopped in Palo Alto for a visit or a meal when he was in the vicinity on business, e.g. Food Machinery Company in San Jose. A great friend and supporter of his sister Lois, he freely gave her advice and words of encouragement.

Holidays such as Easter, July 4th, Thanksgiving, and Christmas were always family gatherings shared with Julian's brother Walter Todd and his wife Ida and son Ted (same age as Doris) and also with Julian's sister Donna and her husband Dr. John McBryan (a dentist who came to America as a young marine engineer from Scotland and received his dental training in San Francisco). The three Todd families gathered for holiday dinners, taking turns in hosting the reunion, each family bringing part of the meal. Often the holiday dinner was in Ione (in the foothills of the Sierras northeast of Lodi near Sutter Creek) where Dr. John McBryan was staff dentist at a state correctional facility and Donna and John had built a lovely home. Most often the holiday dinners were at Seven Pines, the most spacious home of the three. When John retired, he and Donna built a home in Saratoga on Farwell Avenue, near the Pendleton family home where Lois lived as a child. Family holiday gatherings continued in the following years alternating between Palo Alto and Saratoga.

These shared family holidays were always special occasions enjoyed by all with special food, fun, and good fellowship. Both Ida and Donna were home economics (domestic science) teachers and wonderful cooks. A set of verses composed by Julian especially for the occasion (whether he was present or far away) was traditionally shared by family members at the dinner table.

Since Lois worked full-time, the "birthday" child was expected to bake and decorate her or his own cake with the help of siblings and to both plan and prepare the birthday party, beginning around age nine or ten. The success and fanciness of the cake would improve with practice and with the years. By age ten Doris and Elinor were cooking dinner for the family. By age twelve they were planning as well as preparing dinner. When the boys were ten and twelve years of age, they were assigned by their mother the duty of washing and drying dishes. She decided that the boys were old enough to be trusted not to break the dishes and said, "The girls will have plenty of dishes to wash during their lives." Because the girls were preparing meals, the boys now did the dishes.

Lois encouraged all four of her children to participate in after school sports, as she had always participated in athletics. Sports had become an important part of her life and a means of developing and maintaining physical fitness. When after school sports became available in seventh grade, all four children participated each season. The girls went out for soccer, field hockey, volleyball, basketball, softball and swimming; they earned varsity letters in several sports in high school. The boys went out for soccer, baseball and football (James) and became good swimmers.

All four took tennis lessons at the city parks and competed in tennis tournaments. Lois often played tennis with her children until they went off to college, placing her shots with great finesse and skill.

Lois was a serious piano student in her childhood and by high school had become an accomplished pianist. Her sheet music and music books filled the piano bench and the adjacent chest of drawers. So it was not surprising that all four of her children took beginning piano lessons and learned to sight read music. Playing the piano was a great source of enjoyment for Lois and for those who listened to her music. But alas, her busy schedule did not allow much time for playing the piano. It was a rare treat during those busy years when her children were growing up.

All four children began instrumental music at school in the fourth grade. Doris learned to play the clarinet and changed to oboe during junior high, playing in the school orchestra until high school graduation. Elinor learned to play the violin and played in the school orchestra until high school graduation. James played the trumpet, and Hewlett played the accordian. The ensemble of four (quartet) played at family gatherings at Christmas and on other special occasions such as when their father came home for a visit.

CHURCH

In October 1938 when the family first settled in Palo Alto they began attending the small ivy covered, brown shingled First Congregational Church (organized in 1900) on Hamilton Avenue, across from the Post Office in Palo Alto. Lois soon became a member and her children attended Sunday School regularly. As they grew older the girls helped teach Sunday School; they participated in the Pilgrim Fellowship youth group and assumed leadership roles. The girls also sang in the chancel choir. Rev. Augustine Jones was the minister when the family joined the Congregational Church.

As the children approached their teens and became self- conscious about singing their childhood morning blessing at breakfast, it was replaced by a spoken blessing:

> "For this new morning with its light,
> For rest and shelter of the night,
> For rest and food, for love and friends,
> For everything thy goodness sends,
> We thank thee, Heavenly Father."

The next minister was Rev. Arthur Casaday whose paraplegia, due to polio during his college years, necessitated the use of crutches but never limited his participation in activities. Elinor became very active in Pilgrim Fellowship and participated in church camp at Cazadero near Sebastopol for a week every summer. This church involvement gave the youngsters a firm foundation of moral values and helped them to develop a deep personal faith.

The church also provided for Dr. Lois an extended family and a support system which helped give her strength and spiritual renewal for her busy and demanding life. Participation in church was always a time of refreshment and renewal for her and a life-long priority.

Among her favorite scripture passages were Psalms 19, 103 and 121, Isaiah 40: 28 to 31, and Romans 12 (especially verses 9 to 21). She had a deep and vital Christian faith, a calling to service and commitment, and an optimistic and loving spirit. With God's help all things were possible.

When Elinor celebrated her twenty-first birthday during her senior year at Pomona College, the birthday letter she received from her mother included a quote from Alfred Lord Tennyson, "More things are wrought by prayer than this world dreams of."

Elinor and her fiance, Robert M. Christiansen, met at a Labor Day weekend retreat for college students, young adults and professional people at Camp Cazadero. They were married in the little ivy covered First Congregational Church in Palo Alto by Rev. Art Casaday on July 12, 1952. A year later the church property was sold to the city for a parking lot and a new First Congregational Church was built on the edge of town on Embarcadero Road near Newell Road, across from the new Palo Alto City Hall.

In 1942 Mother Pendleton (Jessie Larimore Pendleton) moved from Claremont to Palo Alto into her own small home to be near Lois and under her watchful eye. She died of a stroke in her little home in Palo Alto six years later in 1948. When the new First Congregational Church was built in 1953, Lois designed and made a memorial gift in her mother's memory, a series of clerestory windows the length of the sanctuary containing a variety of pressed leaves and grasses. The leaves were gathered and pressed by Lois and were mounted between two reinforced panes of glass, creating unique windows as beautiful as stained glass windows.

CHILDREN'S EDUCATION

Doctor Lois encouraged each of her four children to pursue educational opportunities to the best of their abilities, to choose accelerated and college preparatory classes, and to participate in extra-curricular activities such as debate and international relations in addition to sports. She considered each child an individual endowed with special talents and with great potential.

Each one was encouraged to develop dreams and goals and to mobilize the time and energy needed to reach those goals. Lois and Julian expected both their daughters and their sons to choose professions (all options were open) and to meet the requirements for their professional training. They promised to provide the tuition money for college and for graduate school for each child. Both Lois and Julian were proud of their children's achievements, being on the honor roll, and entering the colleges and graduate programs of their choice.

Doris won a national Seven College scholarship to Smith College in Northampton, Massachusetts. Following graduation with honors from Smith, she earned her medical degree from Stanford University School of Medicine, becoming a physician like her mother, Lois. Doris had known since her early childhood that this was what she wanted to do.

Elinor studied at Pomona College in Claremont, California, where she pursued a variety of academic interests and majored in pre-med (a broad interdisciplinary major). Her Uncle Morris Pendleton, his wife Gladys, and Aunt Adaline Pendleton had all earned their college degrees at Pomona College. After graduating in 1951, Elinor earned her medical degree from Woman's Medical College of Pennsylvania (Medical College of Pennsylvania) in 1955.

James decided to become an engineer like his father, and studied engineering at Stanford University. After graduation he continued another year earning a Master's degree from Stanford in mechanical engineering.

Hewlett attended Willamette College in Salem, Oregon, as a pre-dental student for one year, then transferred to Cal Poly at San Luis Obispo (California Polytechnic State University) and changed majors. He earned his bachelor's degree in engineering, like his father, and devoted his career to agricultural engineering.

So both daughters followed their mother's career choice and both sons followed their father's career choice. The four children respected and admired their parents and wanted similarly challenging and satisfying lives and careers.

Lois and Julian were excellent role models for their children and were proud of their children's achievements. They taught their children how to work with their hands at hard labor, to persevere, to solve problems, to set goals and achieve, to be responsible, and to enjoy a healthy and vigorous life.

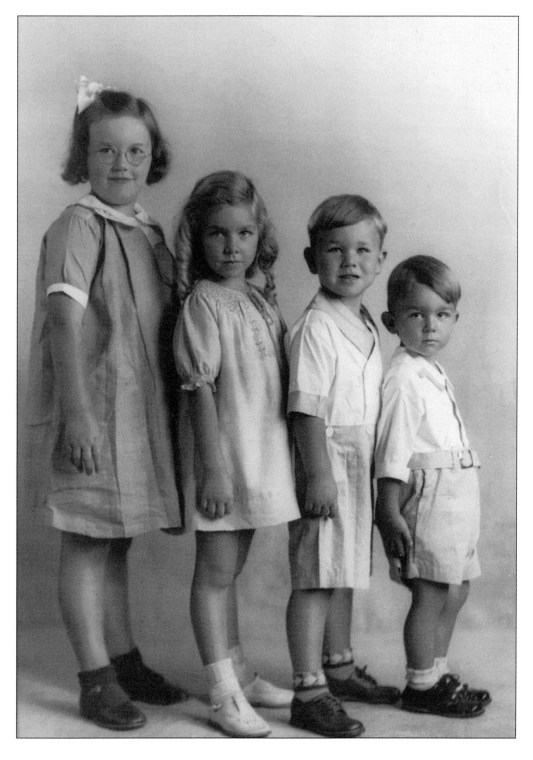

"Stairsteps"—four Todd children: Doris, Elinor, James, and Hewlett—visit America to meet their relatives for the first time in 1935.

CHAPTER 8

Sunset Years

Seven Pines continued to be Lois and Julian Todd's home, even after all four children had married and left the nest. Lois considered the big house a burden to care for and to maintain, but she loved working in her extensive garden. The spacious rose garden was her delight. Another special joy was her garden of gorgeous tuberous begonias and Maidenhair fern under the shade of the sixty foot tall Monterey pines in the spacious front yard. She sprayed her begonias with water by hand every morning and every evening, even after her retirement.

Julian considered their home and garden Paradise after all his years abroad, and he was determined to remain at Seven Pines until his death. He swept the long driveway each morning, raked the leaves, and worked in his wood-yard cutting firewood and making compost. These routines were part of his daily fitness program.

They did indeed continue to live there until they both died, even though it became increasingly dangerous for Lois. Her lack of balance from amyotrophic lateral sclerosis (Lou Gehrig's disease) caused frequent falls. ALS was diagnosed after progressive neurological deficits following her retirement from Stanford.

Julian spent many hours each day in his upstairs study handling his extensive correspondence and other writing, reading, and keeping meticulous household account ledgers. He actively participated in public speaking about China and foreign affairs.

The family returned home often to Seven Pines over the years for birthday celebrations, anniversaries, and holiday gatherings. Doris, David, and their flock of six children who lived nearby in San Bruno, then later in Belmont, came frequently to visit or help with work projects or errands. Hewlett, Sue, and their three children who lived in Morgan Hill, then later in Corning, came often to help with yard work, such as trimming the seven 50 to 60 foot tall pine trees, and other projects. Jim and Ginger and their three children lived in Connecticut for a few years, then Fair Oaks in north central California, and later in Santa Ana, so their visits were infrequent.

Elinor and Bob lived in the east, first in Philadelphia during their years of graduate school, then four years in central Ohio near Columbus in Worthington and Granville. While Elinor was a physician in private practice in Granville two sons were born. They moved to Colorado in 1959 when Bob, a chemical engineer, changed jobs to work for Stearns-Roger Engineering in Denver. They settled in the Denver area and raised three children. Since they were too far from Palo Alto for frequent visits, Lois and Julian would fly to Colorado every year or two, often coming separately. Lois and Julian loved the family outings in the Rocky Mountains and also visited his older brother Alfred and his wife Gertrude in Lamar, Colorado, where Alf had practiced law for 50 years.

Mandatory retirement at age sixty-five forced Dr. Lois Todd to retire in 1960, after 22 years as physician at Stanford University's Student Health Service. She went into private practice part-time after retiring from Stanford, sharing offices with Dr. Masako Baba (lady surgeon who had been classmate of sister Adaline in medical school) and her husband Dr. George Baba (an obstetrician and gynecologist). She continued to practice medicine several years, until increasing neurological deficits prompted her to retire for the second time.

In 1963 a major challenge arose when Hewlett and Sue's youngest child, Joyce, at age 3 became critically ill with a streptococcal infection. Their local physician in Corning, California, treated her with a long-acting sulfonamide. Little Joyce had a severe allergic reaction to the drug, developing Stevens-Johnson syndrome, with sloughing of mucous membranes in all her orifices and sloughing of her skin. Dr. Lois recognized the gravity of the situation, dropped everything and drove to Corning to take charge. She immediately arranged for Joyce to be admitted to Children's Hospital in San Francisco for critical care.

She obtained an ambulance to transport little Joyce to San Francisco, a five hour trip, over two hundred miles. "She rode with Joyce to Children's Hospital in the ambulance. She instructed them not to use the siren and she held Joyce's head, talking to her the entire time, telling her to fight to live," recalled Joyce's mother, Sue.

At Children's Hospital, Joyce was put into strict reverse isolation, which meant that everyone entering her hospital room had to scrub and put on sterile gown, cap, mask, and gloves. Joyce was treated with cortisone, intravenous fluids, and antibiotics to clear up her acute streptococcal infection.

Lois stayed at her granddaughter's bedside day and night to give her encouragement and to watch over her, determined to pull Joyce through her critical condition. The situation remained precarious for four weeks. Much credit for Joyce's recovery goes to her grandmother, Dr. Lois, for her presence and attentive care, and her prayerful concern when Joyce's life was in the balance. "She literally willed Joyce to live," Sue said. "Grandmother Todd's love and care kept Joyce alive against all odds. Always she had faith that Joyce would live." Sue recalled, "When the doctors told me that Joyce had a fifty-fifty chance and I started to cry she (Lois) said, 'Why my dear that's wonderful, when she arrived here she had less than one chance in one hundred'." After four weeks in reverse isolation at Children's Hospital, Joyce was out of danger and had improved sufficiently to return home to Corning to convalesce.

"The strain of caring for Joyce all through those days and nights was so great that Mother Todd's health was never the same," Sue said. "She always lived her life in service for others. She would not have it any other way." Not long after this stress, Lois began to notice increasing weakness in both hands, occasional loss of balance, and some difficulty swallowing. During the next six months various tests were done to determine the cause of the neurological deficits and to rule out multiple sclerosis and muscular dystrophy. After muscle biopsies and several neurological consultations in San Francisco, the diagnosis of amyotrophic lateral sclerosis (Lou Gehrig's disease) was finally confirmed. Lois had noticed hypothenar atrophy along with progressive muscular weakness for several years prior to the definitive diagnosis.

Her busy life continued, although at a slower pace due to her neurological problems. She managed to drive her car, to keep house, care for her garden, and to be as independent as possible. Julian and his sons installed handles in the kitchen for Lois to hold onto while cooking and preparing meals. This was an attempt to reduce the frequency of falls due to her lack of balance. Lois made a padded apron to wear around her hips, decreasing the risk of hip fracture when she fell. Life at home was hazardous because of the many stairs between floors in their home, plus the outside stairs from the ground to the first floor. Added to that challenge were her sense of duty toward fulfilling her household responsibilities and Julian's unwillingness to have help from "strangers" in the house. He would say to Lois impatiently, "You can do it if you just try harder."

Life while traveling was both safer and easier than staying at home. Lois and her husband both enjoyed traveling abroad. Their inquisitiveness prompted them to visit continents and countries they had not seen before, as well as to visit family members living abroad. Fascinated by the world, they were eager to see and learn as much as possible.

Together they enjoyed many interesting trips during their sunset years, even when Lois was disabled: Egypt (from Cairo up the Nile to Aswan Dam); Africa (including wild game preserves, Nairobi, Lake Victoria and Victoria Falls, Lake Tanganyika, Pretoria, Johannesburg, Durban and Cape Town); a railroad tour of South America (from Colombia, Ecuador, and Peru along the Andes, including Machu Picchu, to Bolivia, Chile, Argentina, Brazil, and Venezuela); Hawaii; Alaska; Japan (including a visit with Mitsu, first adopted daughter of Robert and Anne Pendleton); Taiwan (including the fabulous National Chinese Art Gallery); Thailand (including a week with Poonsri, the second adopted daughter of Robert and Anne Pendleton); India, Pakistan (to visit sister Adaline), and Bangladesh; Australia and New Zealand; and Russia. They had hoped to return to China, but it was still closed to American tourists during those years; Nixon's visit to China was the first hint that the doors would open again to Americans.

During each of these trips Lois took detailed notes of what they saw, experienced, and learned. She typed and mailed these descriptive reports to family members after returning home. Julian took colored slides, making a pictorial record of their travels. They enjoyed showing these slides, enriched with observations and insights, to family and friends, and loved reliving their travels. Their last trip to the Orient took place after Lois became so severely disabled with amyotrophic lateral sclerosis that her mobility was markedly impaired and she had to use a wheel chair.

Lois and Julian visited Adaline in Karachi, Pakistan, in the winter of 1967-1968. While Lois remained in Karachi with her sister, Julian explored Pakistan, Afghanistan, and Kashmir. Lois would have enjoyed remaining longer, but Julian insisted on returning to Palo Alto to submit his Internal Revenue Service report on January 15.

When Lois was in Colorado visiting her daughter Elinor, Bob, and their children in May 1967, they decided to purchase a piece of property in Dillon, Colorado. Dillon lies west of the Continental Divide at an elevation of 9,200 feet, about eighty miles west of Denver over Loveland Pass. As the family enjoyed a picnic lunch while overlooking Lake Dillon on Memorial Day, they saw snowflakes in the air; Lois laughed with her family at the refreshing fickleness of weather in Colorado, enjoying every minute. After their picnic the family went to see the property Bob and Elinor wanted to buy as a building site for a mountain cabin.

Lois visited Colorado again the next summer while Bob and Elinor's mountain cabin was under construction in Dillon. Bob pushed Lois in her wheelchair up a temporary ramp into the framed cabin which was not yet enclosed by windows and doors. Lois was thrilled and could imagine how lovely it would be when it was completed. She happily sat in her wheelchair sketching the pine trees outside the open south end of the living room while the family worked on construction projects around her.

While Lois was in Denver with Elinor and family, she wanted to be useful and helpful. She sat at the kitchen table patiently arranging lettuce leaves on the salad plates, even though she was so disabled from ALS she could neither bathe nor dress herself. She used a walker for support and balance. During the days, while Elinor was at work at the Student Health Service at University of Denver, Lois sat at a card table carefully painting an oriental landscape scene from a "paint by number" kit. Elinor would come home to prepare lunch and return to work in the afternoon, while Lois resumed her laborious pursuit of painting the picture, a labor of love. Elinor asked her mother if she would consider staying in Denver, living in their home. Lois replied, "I would love to, but I can't. Your father *needs* me." Her sense of duty and commitment outweighed her self interest and personal safety, even in her final month of life.

That was Lois's last trip to Colorado. Soon after returning home to Palo Alto she deteriorated rapidly; apparently she had sustained a subdural hematoma in one of her frequent falls. During Lois's final illness her daughter Doris phoned Elinor in Denver. She suggested Elinor come home at once as Mother was failing and wanted to see her. When Elinor arrived Mother said to her, "I'm sorry I won't be around to help celebrate your birthday on November 21. Let's plan a special birthday dinner to celebrate your father's birthday on November 1." Doris and Elinor prepared a favorite meal for the family and served it in the dining room. They used the special Coin pattern China from Canton which Lois and Julian had purchased as a wedding gift in 1927. Lois was carried to the table to enjoy this last meal with her family.

At peace with the world, Lois was ready to say good-bye and pass on to her heavenly Father. She died November 11, 1968. Her family buried her ashes in the Pendleton family plot at Madronia Cemetery in Saratoga, California.

RECOLLECTIONS

Sue, her daughter-in-law, recalled, "She was a real mother to me, I was blessed to have had her love and guidance through my young and growing years. She was the most unselfish Christ-like person I have ever known. She was ahead of her time in believing in women's rights. I never received a lecture but in so many ways she guided me. She never interfered and now that my own children are grown I see how hard that is.

"It was important to her that girls be allowed to participate in sports just as boys did. She told me to encourage their interest and not to be concerned about having Tom Boys.

"Once she baby-sat for us when we went to the World's Fair in Washington. We lived in Corning and when we returned she was riding my horse Tom! She galloped down the road and we all laughed; I smile now thinking of her, hair flying. She told me that when she was a young girl she had a pony the color of my horse, a strawberry roan. While she was baby-sitting she also found the time to perform a hysterectomy on our cat!

"She taught me the meaning of sharing. My first Thanksgiving with the Todds was a surprise. Besides all the relatives she always invited several foreign students. By her example she impressed upon me the real meaning of love and sharing.

"She was deeply religious. One of her favorite authors was Harry Emerson Fosdick. She gave me three of his books on prayer and faith. She didn't talk about religion as such, but she lived her life following the teachings of the Bible. One of her favorite prayers was the prayer of St. Francis of Assisi, 'God, make me an instrument of Thy peace.' She told me her favorite bible verse was I Corinthians, chapter 13—she told me to substitute the word love for charity. Hebrews 11:1 was another verse in the Bible that was a favorite.

"When I think of Mother Todd I think of her wonderful sense of humor. Often when she fixed a meal and I helped her we would talk and laugh. She would sometimes laugh until tears would come to her eyes and Grandfather Todd, who would be impatiently sitting at the dining room table, would call, 'Lois, Lois, what's holding things up?' We would have to compose ourselves and stifle our laughs.

"I loved her cooking. Do you remember the wonderful smooth oatmeal cereal she cooked slowly all night? It was so creamy there was none like it. And her creamed chicken, her baked beans and steamed Boston brown bread."

Lois was also known for her wonderful Sunday evening waffle suppers, as well as her home made fruit pies. When family or friends visited she served home made fruit punch, a blend of home canned plum juice and other juices, mid-morning and mid-afternoon with home made cookies or fruit bars. Her date bars were a special favorite with everyone.

Sue reminisced, "I have so many happy memories of her.—She was such a good and loving grandparent to my children. They always loved going to

Grandmother's house.—She was my mother-in-law but she was my mother in the real sense and my most loved friend. She lived her whole life for others. She was the most Christ-like of anyone I've ever known. I miss her in so many ways. I was privileged to know and love her.—Mother Todd lived her life as the Bible teaches us—forgetting oneself and serving others. I feel blessed that for a short time I was able to call her Mother."

QUOTATIONS FROM MEMORIAL RESOLUTION BY THE FACULTY SENATE, STANFORD UNIVERSITY: LOIS PENDLETON TODD (1894-1960)

The following quotations are indications of the respect and high regard in which she was held by her colleagues and friends:

"Lois Todd will always be remembered as a kind, sincere friend who was always willing to give of her time and herself most unselfishly."

"In her relationship to people, whether as doctor, colleague, or friend, she showed unfailing warmth. Her interest was genuine, her sympathy true. Above all she gave of herself."

"Dr. Lois Todd was a physician who considered the students as human beings who needed information about their illnesses. She knew that dispensing medication only is not enough."

"Gave wise counsel and 'motherly care' to both men and women students which carried them through many a difficult academic depression."

"Dr. Lois Todd treated her friends and patients as human beings with deep regard and respect, giving sympathy when needed and bolstering confidence when needed."

"There are those who serve their professions and those who deeply care for individuals as human beings, giving aid and strength to those weak in health—Lois Todd gave both."

"She was highly respected by colleagues of her profession as well as those in academic circles and by those people of the Stanford-Palo Alto community who just 'needed a friend'."

"She was more than just a medical advisor for she deeply cared about the people she met, whether they were private patients, colleagues or students. Foreign students, especially, found in her a sympathetic counselor. She invited many into her home where they were treated as members of the family."

"Dr. Todd was intelligent, kind, gentle and modest. In her quiet way she exemplified the best traditions of personal interest in her students that characterized the early years of Stanford University. An outstanding member of the Stanford Family and a superb physician."

ROLE-MODEL AND MENTOR

Lois Pendleton Todd was an extaordinary woman of vision and sensitivity, strength and courage, commitment and compassion, integrity and humility, graciousness and faith. She welcomed and thrived on adventure and challenge. Her mind was inquisitive and she was highly respected as an astute diagnostician and clinician. She listened to her patients, her family and friends with empathy, intuition, and sensitivity. She was known as a "lateral thinker" and a creative problem solver, as well as a diplomat.

She was a person of action, after thoughtful consideration of what was needed and appropriate, convinced that *actions* speak louder than words. She considered it her responsibilty, even her opportunity, to meet life's demands, whatever they might be. Inspite of all her talents and accomplishments she remained gentle, kind, and humble, always treating others with respect.

Lois believed in a life of service to others. And she was convinced that one person can make a difference in the quality of life, or the health and well-being of another person. This calling is what took her to China in 1920 after completing her medical training. She knew that the needs of the Chinese people for medical care were great, and she felt called to serve them.

Preventive medicine was a primary focus for Lois, long before prevention became popular in our country. She practiced and taught the importance of good nutrition with a balanced diet, including a variety of fruits, vegetables, and whole grains daily. She firmly believed in the importance of daily exercise and physical fitness. Personal hygiene and sanitation, consequences of tobacco and alcohol use, avoidance of excessive sun exposure, adequate sleep, and balance between work and play were other topics she regularly discussed with her patients. During her years as college health physician at Stanford University, her wisdom and counsel made a difference in the lives of many young people. Her enthusiasm, stamina and vigor, optimism and generosity were amazing to all who knew her—her family, her friends, her patients, and her colleagues.

Lois's appreciation of the beauty and wonders of nature gave her great joy. It prompted her to paint, to sketch, and to garden, as well as to support Save the Redwoods League. Her respect for all minorities, her appreciation of diversity, and her compassion for the disadvantaged prompted her to generously support the United Negro College Fund, and to send "care packages" regularly to Mitsu in Japan. She gave generously of her time, talent, and resources to her church. Giving herself brought Lois joy.

She found spiritual renewal through her life-long practice of weekly worship at church. She experienced personal renewal during her twice daily meditation while watering her garden, attending concerts of classical music, or playing the piano. Intellectual renewal came from the practice of medicine and reading medical journals, reading books of a wide variety, and daily discussions of current events during meals with her family and friends.

She served as a wonderful role model and mentor for her children. Periodic reassessment of her priorities at various stages in her life and the life of her family, enabled her to allocate her time and energy effectively. It is no wonder that both of her daughters followed in her footsteps to become physicians, and also chose to marry and to have children. She became an inspiration and beloved friend to all who knew her.

Lois saw her life as an unending journey toward spiritual growth and fulfillment. She was mature and loving, forgiving, accepting and respectful of others, nurturing, and encouraging.

In her sunset years she continued to find joy and zest in the journey of life, learning and participating in every way she could, always wanting to be useful. She grew in knowledge, wisdom and spirit to the very end. Although amyotrophic lateral sclerosis gave her many physical limitations and frustrations, she never complained.

Lois found contentment in memories of a life well-lived, many accomplishments, exciting adventures and many challenges, including her fifty year career as a physician. She found great satisfaction in having successfully raised four children who married and did well in their chosen careers. Her fifteen grandchildren were a great source of joy and hope. She left this world with a sense of fulfillment.

Family Foundations I

New England Roots

MAJOR BRIAN PENDLETON

Brian Pendleton, born in 1599 during the reign of Queen Elizabeth, belonged to the ancient Pendleton family of Manchester, England—several of whom were prominent merchants and churchmen during the 16th century. He married Eleanor Price in 1619 at St. Martin's Church, Birmingham, England. In 1625, a householder in London when Charles I was crowned, he belonged to the parish of "St. Sepulchre's without Newgate." Captain John Smith, adventurer and explorer, was a communicant of this church at the time. Hugh Peters (b. 1598), a lecturer and "apostle of righteousness with reformer's zeal" in this church, emigrated to New England in 1635.

Brian Pendleton, with his wife and children, probably crossed the Atlantic in Governor Winthrop's fleet of eight ships in 1630. They sailed from Southampton to Salem and the mouth of the Charles River (later Boston) settling at Dorchester, Roxbury, and Watertown.

Brian quickly became a leader. In 1634 the first record of Watertown proceedings states three persons were chosen to order civil affairs: William Jennison, John Eddy, and Brian Pendleton. They were known as Selectmen. In 1635 Watertown increased its Selectmen to eleven. Their duties included dividing the land among the inhabitants. Brian Pendleton held at least one public office each year and sometimes held as many as five or six public offices at once.

Some landholders became Freemen, or stockholders in the company, and thus gained a voice in the colony's government. However, Massachusetts and New Haven, Connecticut, in 1631 imposed restrictions on Freemen, requiring them to be church members. Only a fourth of the inhabitants were church members, enabling them to be Freemen with a vote.

In 1635 Watertown decided to limit immigration: 1) no more free land to new arrivals and 2) new arrivals henceforth shall purchase land. Brian Pendleton, who served as a Deputy to the Court of Massachusetts from 1636 to 1638, had to enforce these new rules. Deputies to the Court were chosen by towns. Assistants to the Court were elected by Freemen. During Brian Pendleton's time, the Massachusetts Bay General Court dealt with the following matters:

1. Levy general tax for building stockade around Newtown (Cambridge).

2. Fine or imprisonment for those absent from church services.

3. Banishment of John Smith for "diverse dangerous opinions".

4. Banishment of Roger Williams for antagonism to government ("free thinking and pugnacious").

5. No new churches established without Magistrate approval and approval of majority of elders of existing churches.

6. Empower Freemen to dispose of their own lands, choose their own officers, make such local ordinances as might be necessary.

In 1638 the more liberal inhabitants of Watertown (fifty four families) migrated up the Charles River en route to Concord and established Sudbury. They sold their homes and improved land in Watertown, establishing a new settlement. The local Indian chieftain, Cato (Karte), gave them a deed in 1639. The Pendletons built their home east of the river on Pendleton Hill, now Mt. Pleasant Cemetery.

Sudbury grew quickly. A grist mill was established in 1639 by giving 40 acres of land, frame and planking to a mill operator. In 1640 a church was organized with Edmund Brown as pastor. A meeting house was built in 1643, erected by the householders themselves as a community project. In 1640 the first bridge was built across the river to facilitate commerce in the community.

A "train band" was organized for defense and all able-bodied men were enrolled except magistrates, clergy, and workers in fisheries and ship-building. Weekly military drills were held as well as contests in marksman-ship. Lieutenant Brian Pendleton was one of the founders of the Military Company of Massachusetts, according to the 1648 records. He was appointed by the General Court to drill the military company of Sudbury. He served as Selectman and as Commissioner of Sudbury to 1646, then returned to Watertown where he served as Deputy in 1647 and 1648. He moved to Topsfield, Massachusetts, and served in civil affairs 1648 and 1649.

Next he moved to Portsmouth, New Hampshire, where he was appointed Associate Justice from 1651 to 1665. He also served as Selectman from 1652 to 1662 and Commissioner and Commander of the military company. He was also selected as Justice at Kittery, Maine. He served on the "annexation commission" to Maine from Massachusetts and was Deputy to the General Court of Massachusetts from 1653 to 1663. He was town treasurer of Portsmouth from 1654 to 1663.

After giving his goods, houses, warehouses, wharves, and lands in Portsmouth, New Hampshire, Westerly, Rhode Island, and Sudbury, Massachusetts, to his son James, Brian Pendleton moved to Winter Harbor (Saco), Maine, in 1665 where he was chosen Selectman 1666 and 1667, elected a Burgess to General Court of the Province of Maine in 1667, appointed surveyor of highways, served as Major of York County regiment in 1668, Associate Justice of the Province of Maine 1668 to 1676, town clerk of Saco in 1672, and assessor of taxes at Saco in 1676, and became deputy president of the Province of Maine in 1680.

He returned to Portsmouth in 1676 with his wife because of the Indian War. He remained in Portsmouth 1677 to 1678 then returned to Saco to review the devastation wrought by the Indians. He died the winter of 1680-1681 at the age of 81.

Brian Pendleton was an active and energetic man, acquisitive and generous, devout and pragmatical in every sense of the word with a long career in public affairs. He was somewhat inclined toward liberality in his earlier days, but later became an ardent partisan, a typical Puritan, and engaged in enforcing the laws. He became involved in maintaining authority over the non-Puritan settlements which Massachusetts absorbed "at the Eastward"—Portsmouth, New Hampshire, and Maine. During these years he became engaged in foreign commerce by sailing ships, including exporting timber and importing rum and sugar from Barbados.

CAPTAIN JAMES PENDLETON

James Pendleton, the son of Brian Pendleton, was born in London, England, in 1627 or 1628. His parents emigrated to New England before he was six years old, settling in Watertown, Massachusetts, before 1634. They lived in Sudbury, Massachusetts, from 1639 to 1646. James was the only son of Brian Pendleton to leave descendents. His parents deeded their homestead in Sudbury plus 140 acres to James in 1656-1657. James Pendleton married Mary Palmer in 1647. She died in 1655 after bearing three children: James (1650), Mary (1653) and Hannah (1655). They all lived in Sudbury, Massachusetts. In 1656 James married Hannah Goodenow (age 16) who bore him eight children: Brian (1659), Joseph (1661), Edmund (1665), Ann (1667), Caleb (1669), Sarah (1675), Eleanor (1679), and Dorothy (1686). James and Hannah lived in

Portsmouth after their marriage. James served as grand juryman of Portsmouth, New Hampshire, in 1659; constable in 1661; town clerk 1663 and 1664; Selectman 1663 to 1668; local magistrate (Commissioner) 1667-1671; Captain of the military company 1666 to 1674 and was one of nine men to establish the first Congregational Church in Portsmouth, New Hampshire, in 1671.

He moved his family in 1674 to 700 acres in Westerly, Rhode Island (or Stonington, Connecticut), east of the Pawcatuck River, which his father had deeded him in 1666. Whether this land belonged to Rhode Island or to Connecticut was under dispute for many years.

War with the Indians (King Philip's War) against the Pequots erupted soon after James and his family arrived. The war lasted two years and involved the Wampanoags and Narragansetts as well as the Pequots. There were many captives, including women and children, being sold as slaves.

James was active in the first Congregational Church in Stonington, Connecticut. He was elected Selectman of Stonington from 1677 to 1679. Since his property was east of the Pawcatuck River he was required in 1679 as a resident of Rhode Island to swear to a loyalty oath to the King of England and the Colony of Rhode Island. In 1686 James became a Freeman of Westerly, Rhode Island, and also was elected Selectman in 1686. He was appointed Justice in the Court of Kingstown in 1686 and of the King's Province in 1688 at Newport, Rhode Island.

James was clearly following in his father's footsteps in assuming numerous civil responsibilities. While living on his 700 acres in Westerly, Rhode Island, as Freeman he was elected Selectman in 1686 and 1691; moderator of Town Meeting 1687, 1688 and 1700; purchased 1000 acres at Watch Hill (Pawcatuck Neck also known as Squomacutt) in 1689; tax assessor 1699; town councilman 1699, 1701 to 1704 and 1705 to 1710. He gave thirty acres of Watch Hill estate to his daughter Eleanor in April 1709 for her love and kindness during his sickness. He died in Westerly in 1709 at the age of 81 or 82. He was buried in the old cemetery on the point of land running into Pawcatuck River known as "Graves Neck", south of Lottery Village (now Avondale).

(ENSIGN) JOSEPH PENDLETON

Joseph Pendleton was born in Sudbury, Massachusetts, on Dec. 29, 1661. He was the son of Capt. James Pendleton and his second wife, Hannah Goodenow. He moved with his family to Westerly, Rhode Island, in 1674 at age 12. At age 17 he took the oath of allegiance to the King of England and the Colony of Rhode Island at Westerly on Sept. 17, 1679 along with his father. He was chosen to be tax assessor in 1695, constable in 1697, and town clerk in 1701.

Joseph married Deborah Minor on July 8, 1696; their daughter Deborah was born Aug. 29, 1697, and Joseph's wife died ten days later on Sept. 8, 1697. He married Patience Potts on Dec. 11, 1700 who bore him three sons: Joseph 1702, William 1704, and Joshua 1706. Joseph Pendleton became a Freeman June 22, 1699; he owned 100 acres. He was a farmer with cattle, he made cheese, grew corn, barley, wheat, flax, oats, hay, and fodder.

At age 45 at the time of his death (Sept. 18, 1706) his estate included two oxen, ten cows, six yearlings, three steers, one bull, seven calves, 23 sheep, 12 swine, and a hive of bees.

COLONEL WILLIAM PENDLETON

William Pendleton was born in Westerly, Rhode Island, March 23, 1704. He was the second of three sons of Joseph Pendleton and his second wife, Patience Potts. William was baptized in the Congregational Church on May 28, 1704. He was one of the council which formed the Church of Christ in 1742. He became a Deacon in 1752. He was a justice of the peace, served as a representative in the General Assembly of Rhode Island, and was a Major in the Third Regiment of King's County militia. He became Colonel in 1750 and served as muster master in the French and Indian War. William was president of Westerly Town Council 1762 to 1781 (member of town council 1757-1781). He raised soldiers for the Revolutionary War.

William married Lydia Burrows of Groton, Connecticut, (b. 1703) on March 10, 1725. They had nine children: William, Amos, Freelove, Lydia, Peleg, John, Benjamin, Joshua and Ephraim. Lydia, William's wife, died in Westerly, Rhode Island, in August 1750. William Pendleton married his second wife, Mrs. Mary Chesebrough (widow) on April 4, 1751. There were four children by this marriage, two sons and two daughters: Nathan, Keturah, Lucy, and Isaac (who drowned at age twenty).

William Pendleton was a farmer in 1728, raising cattle and horses, and was a Freeman of Westerly, Rhode Island. He became inspector of commodities in 1734 to 1744 and was juryman 1734, 1743, and 1754. He was Deputy to the Rhode Island General Assembly in 1746. William Pendleton had an excellent reputation for fairness and square dealing. He served as head of Westerly Town Council from 1762 to 1781, a total of nineteen years. He died in Westerly, Rhode Island, on August 23, 1786 at age 82.

LIEUTENANT PELEG PENDLETON

Peleg Pendleton was born in Westerly, Rhode Island, on July 9, 1733, one of seven sons and two daughters born to Col. William Pendleton and his first wife Lydia Burrows. Peleg began going to sea at an early age. All nine sons of Col. William Pendleton (seven by his first marriage and two by his second marriage) became master mariners. By age 29, in 1762, Peleg was part owner of the schooner *Dolphin*. On Sept. 7, 1758 he married Ann Park at Westerly, Rhode Island. They had eleven children (six sons and five daughters): Peleg, Jr. (who died as a young man), Thomas, twins William and Joseph, Green, Phineas, Anna, Abigail (who died age 5), twins Lydia and Abigail 2nd, and Prudence. All five sons who reached adulthood became master mariners like their father. The daughters married mariners. Peleg was a master mariner of great renown.

"Peleg Pendleton must have been among those afflicted (with smallpox) at some time in his early life for in 1774 we find he had been delegated to care for those then in the Westerly smallpox hospital." Peleg was in charge of procuring provisions for the victims of smallpox as well as responsible for their confinement and the enforcemnt of the quarantine.

In 1775 Peleg was deeded 250 acres of land in Maine near Penobscot Bay where he cleared land and built a log cabin between 1773 and 1775. The land was near Fort Pownal (now Fort Point), a trading post frequented by French fur traders and Indians. The town established later south of his land was named Prospect, now called Searsport, Maine. Peleg, Jr. (b. 1760) went with his father to Maine and stayed to protect the deeded acres while his father returned to Westerly to get the family. However the Revolutionary War broke out and eight years elapsed before Peleg moved his family to Maine in 1783. When Peleg returned to his land near Fort Pownal no trace of Peleg, Jr., could be found, his son having vanished sometime between 1775 and 1783. Peleg was elected Lieut. of Capt. Babcock's Artillery on June 3, 1777. He was the 64th signer of the "Test Act" in 1776 in Westerly, Rhode Island, pledging allegiance to the new government of the colonies.

"Like his older brother Amos, Peleg Pendleton was the progenitor of a spendid race of master mariners, those vigorous and self reliant men who in the palmy days of American shipping carried our flag on all the seven seas."

Lieut. Peleg Pendleton lived with his family in Searsport, Maine, from the end of the Revolutionary War until his death July 10, 1810, at age 77. His grave is on Pendleton family land which was given to Searsport for a cemetery and is now known as Bowditch Cemetery (probably named after the famed New England navigator, Nathaniel Bowditch).

CAPTAIN PHINEAS PENDLETON

Phineas Pendleton was born in Stonington, Connecticut, (Westerly, Rhode Island) on September 26, 1780, son of Lieut. Peleg Pendleton and his wife Ann Park. Phineas became a master mariner like his father and four

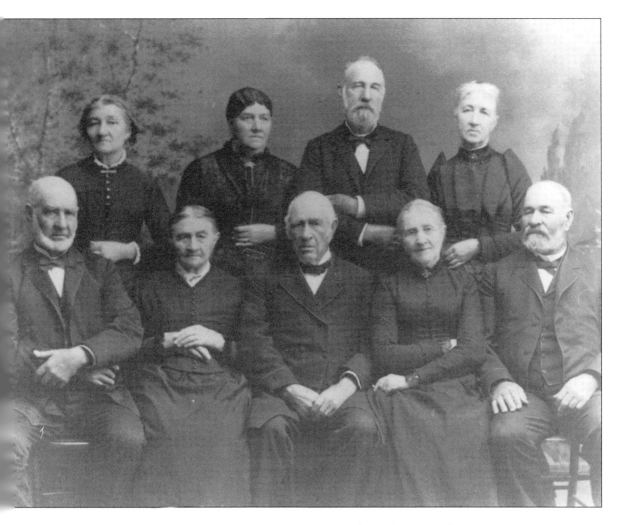

Pendleton family of Searsport, Maine in 1890. John Gilmore Pendleton (1828-1899), paternal grandfather of Lois, at far right.

brothers. He married Nancy Gilmore (b. 1788) of Belfast, Maine, on March 28, 1805. They had six sons and six daughters of whom eleven reached adulthood and all lived in Searsport or Belfast, Maine. The five sons who reached adulthood all became sea captains (master mariners). Of the six daughters, four married sea captains and two remained single. In 1886 a family picture was taken of their nine surviving children on the 80th birthday of Phineas, Jr.: James Gilmore (1828-1899), Phineas, Jr. (1806-1896), John Gilmore (1828-1899), Benjamin Franklin, Mary, Nancy, Esther, Prudence, and Maria Emilene. Nathan (1808-1880) and Margaret died before the picture was taken.

Son Phineas, Jr. (b. Aug. 1806, d. July 1896) was a sea captain commanding over twenty large sailing vessels which he sailed all over the world.

In 1844, as Captain of the Searsport brig *John Carver*, he brought a pair of Hereford cattle into Maine, the start of that breed in the New England States.

John Gilmore Pendleton, the third son, was born November 8, 1828, in Searsport, Maine, and became a master mariner as did all of his brothers.

Capt. Phineas Pendleton was captured by the British during the War of 1812. The records of the Vice Admiralty Court in Halifax, Nova Scotia, have the following item in regard to his capture by the British: "*Schooner Belfast* 124 tons, P. Pendleton, master, bound for Penobscot in ballast, captured 7 April, 1813, by privateer *Retaliation*."

Phineas Pendleton was commissioned Captain in the 2nd Regiment Infantry, 1st Brigade, 10th Division, Massachusetts Militia, June 11, 1813. He received pay for service at Belfast, Maine, Sept. 2-21, 1814. He died at Searsport, Maine, Feb. 26, 1873, at age 93. His grave is in the same cemetery as his father Peleg's in Searsport, Maine.

CAPTAIN JOHN GILMORE PENDLETON

John Gilmore Pendleton was born in Searsport, Maine, on Nov. 8, 1828, the son of Capt. Phineas Pendleton and his wife, Nancy Gilmore of Belfast, Maine. He went to sea early and became a master mariner calling at many foreign ports. He was Captain of nine large vessels (including bark, ship and brig) during his career and part owner of many. John Gilmore Pendleton was Captain of the following vessels:

> Bark: *John Gardner* 1852
> Ship: *Gace Ross* 1859
> Ship: *William H. Connor* 1877, 1885-86, 1893-94
> Ship: *Henry B. Hyde* 1888
> Brig: *Leghorn*
> Brig: *Kentucky*
> Ship: *Borodino*
> Ship: *Nancy Pendleton*
> Ship: *Lewis Walsh*

John Gilmore Pendleton married Mary Ann Pendleton, daughter of cousin Green Pendleton, Jr., on Sept. 5, 1849. She traveled with him abroad, as was common for the wives and children of sea captains of Searsport, and died in Cronstadt, Russia, on Sept. 16, 1853. He married Sarah E. Blanchard of Belfast, Maine, on April 20, 1856. The two children by his first wife died in infancy, but by the second he had three sons and three daughters. The youngest son died in childhood, the other two, Charles Shepherd and John Louis Pendleton, raised families. The daughters' names after marriage were Evelyn Morrison, Martha Jackson, and Edith DuBose.

The ship *William H. Connor* was a "Down Easter", a square rigger built in Searsport, Maine, in 1877 with twelve square sails and three fore and two aft jibs. Tonnage: 1496 tons. Dimensions: length 210 feet, beam 40 feet, depth 24 feet. Master Builder: Marboro Packard. Cost: $110,000 (sixty four shares, sixteen shares owned by Pendletons). This was the last and largest square rigger built in Searsport, Maine. Trade: brought lumber from Maine to Liverpool and coal from England to China around Cape Horn.

The ship *Henry B. Hyde* was a "Down Easter" (square rigger) built in Bath, Maine. In 1888 Capt. John Gilmore Pendleton sailed this ship from San Francisco to Honolulu in ten days (averaging 288 miles per day), setting a speed record for sailing ships.

Phineas Pendleton III (grandson of Phineas and nephew of John Gilmore), born in 1831, was also a successful master mariner as were his father and grandfather. "His wife accompanied him on many of his voyages, particularly in the *Henry B. Hyde* which was launched at Bath, Maine, in November 1884. Its length of 269 feet made it one of the biggest wooden ships ever launched in this country, and it was well adapted to take the wife and the children of Captain Pendleton on his long trips. The first one, around Cape Horn, was followed by six others around the stormy point of land." Three of his younger children, a daughter and two of his sons, died in South America in 1869 from cholera in the Galapagos Islands off the coast of Peru.

John Gilmore Pendleton, master mariner renowned for his speed record in the *Henry B. Hyde*, died in Everett, Massachusetts, on April 23, 1899, at the age of 71 years.

JOHN LOUIS PENDLETON

John Louis Pendleton was born in Searsport, Maine, on July 24, 1866, the son of John Gilmore Pendleton, master mariner, and his second wife, Sarah E. Blanchard of Belfast, Maine. He was one of three sons and three daughters by this marriage. The first son of this second marriage was named Charles Shepherd and the second son John Louis. The youngest son died in childhood.

The era of great sailing ships was over, as steam ships had been invented and successfully competed with sailing vessels for cargo transport to foreign ports. After the Civil War, steel hull steam-driven ships or "tramp steamers", came into common use. Sea captains became merchants of durable goods, hardware and ship chandlery. Thus John Louis Pendleton entered the hardware business and became involved with selling tools, and later in his life the manufacture

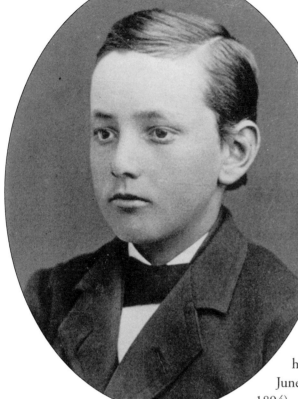

John Louis Pendleton of Searsport, Maine, age 10 in 1876.

of tools. During his childhood in Searsport, Maine, sea captains were jokingly referred to as "Maine-iacs."

His first job was in a hardware store in Belfast, Maine. He moved west at age 21 to work in the Morrison Hardware Co., which was owned by his sister Evelyn Morrison's husband, in Minneapolis, Minnesota. He married Jessie Larimore, a young school teacher who was the daughter of Dr. Andrew Jackson Larimore of Bryan, Ohio (near Toledo), and his widow Mrs. Adaline Ann (Morris) Moore Larimore of Minneapolis, on June 25, 1889. John Louis and Jessie had five children: Robert Larimore (b. June 25, 1890) and Lois (b. April 14, 1894) were born in Minneapolis; Morris Blanchard (b.Feb. 4, 1901) and David Andrew (b. Aug.21, 1909; d. 1914) were born in Saratoga, California; and Adaline (b. Feb. 7, 1917) was born in Berkeley, California.

In 1895 he moved west to Saratoga, California, with his wife and two small children, Robert Larimore (b. June 25, 1890) and Lois (b. April 14, 1894). They settled on ten acres of land which they planted with prune trees (a "prune ranch") a mile south of Saratoga along the west side of Santa Clara valley, a region known for its fruit orchards: prunes, apricots, pears, cherries, and grapes.

J. Louis worked as a traveling hardware salesman, prune rancher, and also county supervisor of roads. The family thrived and prospered in Saratoga and lived there for 18 years. In 1913 the family moved to Berkeley, California, where Robert and Lois were undergraduate and graduate students at the University of California.

When J. Louis became a partner in Plomb Tool Company he moved to Los Angeles. The family followed in 1918 when Morris graduated from Berke-

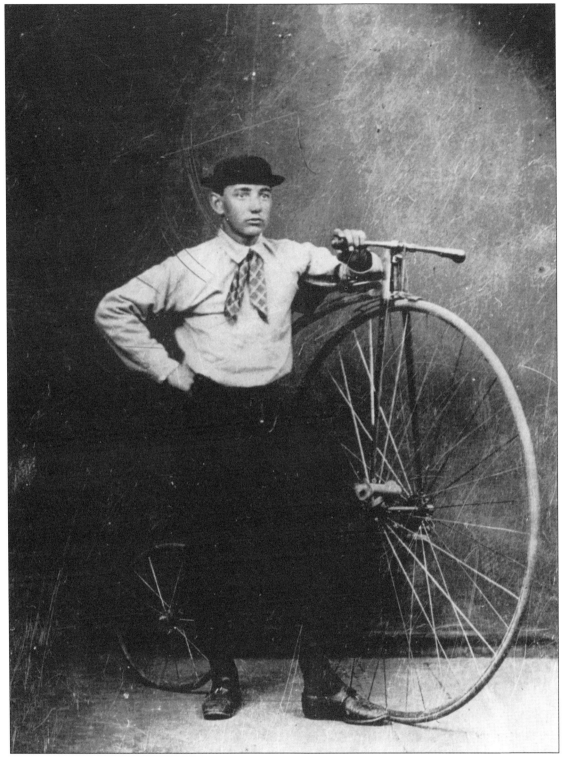

John Louis Pendleton age 20 with bicycle.

ley High School. John Louis died unexpectedly in Los Angeles at age 57 on April 7, 1924, from a mastoid infection and pneumonia following a business trip.

John Louis Pendleton's ashes were buried at the foot of the magnificent Madronia tree in the family plot he had purchased many years earlier in Saratoga, next to his son David who had died of diphtheria at age 5. Louis was a quiet, thoughtful, serious, energetic and hard working family man with a sense of humor. He enjoyed investing in mountain property, primarily because he was a conservationist and wanted to save magnificent trees and scenic mountain drives from the destruction of future development. He wanted to preserve the beauties of nature for future generations.

Pennsylvania Roots

WILLIAM MORRIS

William Morris was a shoemaker and a farmer, born Dec. 11, 1793 in Uniontown, Fayette County, Pennsylvania. Uniontown is located in southwest Pennsylvania about 15 miles from West Virginia. He was a Welshman with a taste for politics, poetry, and religion. Cousin Mary Embleton, retired school teacher, wrote in her lengthy memoirs of her grandfather, "His forbears were probably Virginians who came into western Pennsylvania by way of the Braddock Trail" sometime before his birth. William's mother was Rebecca Boone.

"Western Pennsylvania was still the frontier in 1793. The Indians were being pushed back as far as Indiana, the forests had been partially cleared, fields were fenced and yielded a variety of food besides wool and flax for clothing. The log houses were weather-proof and consisted usually of more than one room with even the occasional luxury of glass windows. It was a so-called subsistence economy with very little money and much economic cooperation." Activities included corn husking and barn raisings, quilting parties, and fulling parties—"where the men tread with bare feet in soapy water the newly woven blankets". William Morris told a story from his childhood about watching maple sap boil through the night, alone in the forest. The memory of prowling Indians and wild beasts was still fresh; men who had experienced these terrors still lived.

"The farmers of southwestern Pennsylvania were not illiterate frontiersmen. They were alive to the problems of their day and jealous of their rights. In 1788 they had met in Uniontown to demand that a Bill of Rights be embodied in the Constitution before Pennsylvania ratified it. About the time William Morris was born they had resisted the taxation of their stills, because they thought the seaboard business men were treating them unfairly. Although they were forced to submit, their interests were afterwards more carefully considered."

"A few of these men were highly educated. The most important was Albert Gallatin, who although of a noble and wealthy Swiss family, had come to America to further the ideology of democracy. He settled near Uniontown where he had a gun and a glass factory. At the time of which we are writing he was Secretary of the Treasury (under President Thomas Jefferson) and spent little time in Fayette County, but the influence of such a man permeates a community and remains long after he has left. Uniontown was devoted to the ideas of Gallatin and Jefferson. All his life William Morris was a liberal in politics, a Jeffersonian Republican, a Democrat, and after 1856 a Republican."

"In religion he leaned toward mild skepticism. He would not allow his daughters to attend revivals and camp meetings. He believed that to love God and thy neighbor was the essence of Christianity. He did not favor dancing and was strictly against card playing. Above all he was original and independent in his thinking and tolerant of the beliefs of others."

When he was eighteen, August 27, 1812 he enlisted in Captain Thomas Collins' Company of Pennsylvania Volunteers; he served until September 18, 1813 as a private during the War of 1812. At the end of this tour of duty, he re-enlisted and was in the battle of Chippewa, and served to the end of that war. "In August 1812, when William Morris volunteered as a private, eighteen years old and untrained, he was to help hold the line of Lake Erie and the Maumee River under General Harrison. In that same month Detroit and Chicago had surrendered to the British. That left Ohio exposed to the Indians, who had promised to fight for the British. The Virginians and Pennsylvanians started north through eastern Ohio toward Sandusky. They were to meet the troops from Kentucky and Ohio at the rapids of the Maumee where Harrison planned to concentrate his troops and supplies for an advance on Detroit. However wet weather interfered with the plans and bogged down the troops and supplies. Harrison had to come back from Maumee in late October to round up his men. The idea of an easy capture of Detroit had to be abandoned. In January the ground finally froze and men and supplies were rushed to Fort Meigs (near Toledo) or to the mouth of the Sandusky on Lake Erie. In May, Fort Meigs withstood a heavy seige and Harrison moved to protect the building of ships for Perry."

William re-enlisted, probably in the 22nd Regiment of the regular infantry which was made up of men from Pennsylvania and Virginia, to take part in the Chippewa battle. To keep control of Lake Erie and prevent an invasion of New York State, General Brown crossed the Niagara River with an army

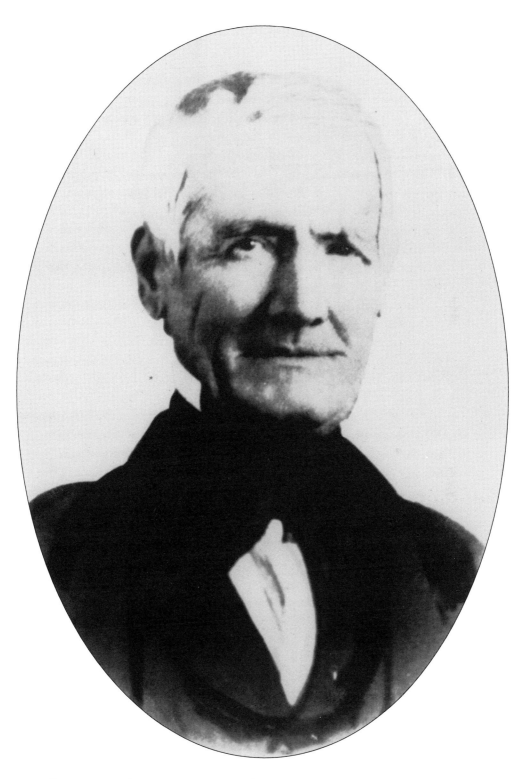

William Morris (1793-1861), maternal great grandfather of Lois Pendleton.

of 3500 regulars, volunteers, and Iroquois Indians in July 1814. He captured Fort Erie and hastened to meet the British at Chippewa, near Navy Island below the Falls. The brigade under Winfield Scott led the way and arrived July 5, numbering about 1300. They marched across the river and advanced, firing rapidly, at an oblique angle. The British broke and crumbled although they numbered 1800. Henry Adams wrote, "Small as the affair was and unimportant in military results, it gave to the American army a pride and character it had never before possessed."

William was mustered out sometime in 1815 after the peace had been concluded. According to the law he received $128 and a warrant for 320 acres of land on the frontier (for William the dank forests of northwestern Ohio, west of Toledo).

The Braddock Road was now widened and surfaced at federal expense and was named the Cumberland Road. This was the first national road, established by an act of Congress in 1806 at the behest of Albert Gallatin, who owned land near Uniontown. It ran from Baltimore and Washington through Uniontown and on to the Mississippi. It was congested by emigrants and "freighters" (Conestoga covered wagons) going west.

When William Morris returned home from the wars, he found little need for a shoemaker; people could buy better-looking shoes at the general store. William moved to Maiden Creek, Berks County, in eastern Pennsylvania, just north of Reading. The beautiful, fertile valley of the Schulkyll River had been farmed by Quakers and German Pietists for over a hundred years. He married Hannah Smith, age eighteen, in 1819 and stayed in Maiden Creek until 1835. Hannah's father was a blacksmith from Maryland. Her mother was Catherine Miller who was of German or Pennsylvania Dutch descent and had a very strong character.

William and Hannah were a handsome couple and were hard-working and thrifty, for by 1835 they had saved enough to buy a farm in Ohio and pay the expenses of moving and stocking. Their move may have been influenced by the school election of 1834 for free public schools. The Quakers and Pennsylvania Dutch Pietists had their own sectarian schools. William wanted free public schools for his children. Discussions over the school issue became so bitter in the eastern part of the state that people refused to speak or do business with those who favored free schools. In Berks County the measure was lost by a 3 to 30 vote but it was carried unanimously in Fayette County.

Seven children were born to William and Hannah in Maiden Creek: Lewis S. Morris (January 1820), Rebecca Morris (August 1821), Mary S. Morris (September 1824), John Milton Morris (February 1826), Benjamin Franklin

Morris (August 1829), Catherine S. Morris (January 1832) and Isaac B. (May 1834 to 1850).

When William Morris and his family moved to Ohio in 1835 his brother Lewis Morris, mother-in-law, Catherine Miller Smith, and her daughter Mary Smith (Aunt Polly), and his brother-in-law Lewis Smith with wife and children moved with him, lock, stock, and household gear. They traveled in Conestoga wagons on the Cumberland Road so that they passed through Uniontown, where they stopped to visit relatives. Frank remembered that his father took him over to West Virginia to visit a brother who had a fine farm and beautiful horses.

They settled in Paris Township, Stark County, Ohio, a rolling fertile country in east central Ohio, already cleared. The post-office was New Franklin about fifteen miles east of Canton. William soon built a substantial two-story house, a barn, a spring-house, a brick oven, and a shop where he made and mended shoes of the family and perhaps others. When he became justice of the peace, he used the shop for that activity.

Four more daughters were born after the family reached Ohio: Rachel Jane (1836), Adaline Ann (1839), Sarah G. (1841), and Theodosia Rosamond (1844). Mary chose the name for the youngest sister as she was "tired of old-fashioned Mary, Jane and Sarah". The family treasured affectionate baby names and the youngest daughter was known as Dosia (Dosha).

Soon after arriving in Ohio, William began a campaign for a district school. In Ohio a share of the expense was born by the Federal government from a fund set aside for that purpose in the Northwest Ordinance. There was much opposition from tax-conscious farmers like Lewis Smith, his brother-in-law. William Morris won and the school was built, a small log house with backless benches. The teacher had a raised seat and a knife for making quill pens. The older children attended in the winter, the younger children in the summer. In their home there was always an interest in books and schooling. Jane remembered that the children were lined up at night to recite to their father long poems and passages from orations. When McGuffey's readers came they were a great source of declamation: "Give me liberty or give me death."

Hannah bore and nursed the children, cooked the meals by the open hearth, dipped the candles from lard and tallow, made the soap, prepared the flax and wool for spinning, spun and wove them into cloth, and made them into clothes for the family. Grandmother knit the stockings and father made the shoes. Hannah and her girls were all dressed in homespun "linsy-woolsy", all alike except that the little girls wore shorter skirts and pantalets (tube-like affairs of linen tied over the knees).

During the early years on the farm in Ohio, the family could not afford to buy dishes, so Hannah made buckwheat cakes each meal and laid them on the table at each place to serve as a plate. Food was served on the buckwheat cakes. When the children finished eating their food, they ate their buckwheat cakes, and the table was wiped off clean; no dishes to wash or put away.

"Mary bathed the four little girls each Saturday night in front of the fire. Then she put on their linen chemises (shimmies) which served as nightgowns and undergarments all week. She chased them up to bed, and seizing each squealing child by the shimmie-tail swung her twice before throwing her into the corn-husk bed. Toys were almost unknown. Jane and Adaline made dolls of crooked-neck squash." A rag doll was a special treat.

When William Morris sold his wheat in Canton he would bring a few treats to the children such as a few "sugar sticks". Once when the price of grain was uncommonly high, he bought two calico parasols for Adaline and Jane. These were kept with great care and finally used in public for the Fourth of July parade in Paris. The children were invited to march in the parade. Dressed in their best they walked to Paris and waited with the other children. Then the "marshall" announced the the girls dressed in white should go first. The Morris girls were the only ones in colored clothes (they did not own any white clothes). Jane said, "Let's not march." But Kate said, "We will too. We'll not stay out." So they stepped proudly at the very end of the procession, their heads held high under their calico parasols.

William was a kind father with a sense of humor, interested in education for his daughters as well as his sons. He himself had hungered for schooling which only the well-to-do could afford in his youth. In his second son, Milton, he saw one who would fulfill his desires and dreams. The boy loved to study, eagerly lapped up all that the district schools could give, and taught himself Latin and Greek. William Morris could not afford to send his son to a private academy. Fortunately a truly remarkable Yankee school-master named Alfred Holbrook came to Ohio.

This man devoted his long life (1816 to 1909) to teaching, especially to the training of country teachers. Enthusiastic and dedicated, he always offered instruction and living expenses at the lowest price possible. Milton went to him to study. Forty years later another young student of Alfred Holbrook was Cordell Hull. In his Memoir (Vol. I, 22,23), Cordell Hull wrote, "The normal schools founded by Professor Holbrook gave splendid instruction—I studied higher mathematics including calculus, advanced rhetoric, which covered all the best phases of literature, and some of the sciences. There I took part in strenuous discussion held by the school's debating societies. Students were from many states both north and south, and a fine fellowship and comradeship sprang up among all alike."

The railroad had come to Ohio, and William Morris was prompt in taking his first ride. He bought a ticket, entered the baggage car and sat on a trunk until the brakeman arrived and said, "Sir, you will be more comfortable in the coach." To which William replied, "Sir, I thank you, I am quite comfortable where I am."

CATHERINE MILLER SMITH

William's mother-in-law, Catherine Miller Smith, was a colorful, strong character. She came to Ohio with her son and two daughters, but not to live with them as a proper grandmother. She bought a farm on a hill near her married children and worked the farm herself with the help of her unmarried daughter, Mary Smith (Aunt Polly), and the grandsons, especially Frank. Besides managing her farm, she kept all her children and grandchildren in stockings and was perpetually knitting new ones and footing old ones. Her thrift was excessive. She was a sturdy little woman, broad in the hips. She had great endurance and stamina and lived until over ninety. It was told that one icy, bitter cold day, a neighbor half her age came to visit her. When she left, old Catherine bundled herself up, took her cane and went down the slippery hill to make sure her guest had not fallen and hurt herself.

Aunt Polly was Hannah's older sister and as dearly loved by the Morrises as their mother. She worked for them as needed, listened to them, comforted them and loved them. While William lived she was sure of protection but when he died and the family scattered, her fate was sad indeed. Catherine Smith willed her farm to her son Lewis, who was even more avaricious than she and neglected Aunt Polly.

TYPHOID OUTBREAK

In 1850 the Morris family seemed thriving. Lewis, Rebecca, and Mary were married. Milton was teaching and attending Normal School, Kate was looking forward to school also, when a tragedy befell New Franklin. David Miller, the enterprising young merchant and husband of Rebecca, went to Philadelphia and came home sick with typhoid fever. The wells were soon poisoned, and every family in the neighborhood was affected. In January, William Morris lost his oldest son, Lewis, and his youngest son, Isaac, within two weeks. All the children were very sick. In the midst of this trouble Dr. McCarthy rode in one night, his baby wrapped in his cloak. Mary, his wife and William and Hannah's second daughter, had just died in childbirth. Hannah undertook the care of the newborn baby in addition to all her other labors. When all survivors were out of danger, Hannah died March 14, 1850. Aunt Polly was a wonderful help and comfort to the four younger girls.

Jane was nearly fourteen. Unwilling to show her grief at her mother's death, she held back her tears until milking time, when she pressed her head against the cow's smooth, warm flank and cried her grief out. But it was Kate upon whom the burden of labor and responsibility fell heaviest. She was eighteen and eager for more education. She had to care for her father, Frank and the four younger sisters, and the little baby. They had no facilities for feeding him. Jane remembered wrapping a rag around a quill to serve as a nipple to a bottle of cow's milk. Even so little Willie McCarthy lived for more than a year; then he too died.

William Morris hired a neighbor woman to do the heaviest work. He was now able to buy things once made by Hannah such as cloth. Still soap making, and candle making, and the huge washings to do without washboard or wringer remained as chores. Jane was headstrong, Addie a little lazy, so Kate appealed to her brother Milton to write and advise the younger sisters regarding their behavior. He did so with tact and effectiveness.

Just as Milton seemed most promising as a teacher and helpful to his family, he died. The last item in his diary, dated July 5, 1851, was "Now, ho for a ride on Alexander the Great." The horse, high spirited, bolted back into the stable through a low door; Milton was killed instantly. The whole family suffered the loss, but especially William Morris.

He had one remaining son, Benjamin Franklin, or Frank, the kind and faithful, efficient farmer. He wished to marry and have a farm of his own, so William gave him the warrant for the land that was due him for service during the War of 1812. The land was in the northwestern corner of Ohio, in the undrained heavy forest. Frank cleared and drained the land at a heavy cost of labor and life. His first wife and one of his children died. He lived there near Bryan, Ohio, the rest of his life.

ADALINE ANN MORRIS

Adaline was born in 1839 in New Franklin, Paris Township, Stark County, Ohio to William Morris and his wife, Hannah, four years after the family moved west. Her mother died of typhoid in 1850 when Adaline was thirteen. Her older sister Kate wanted more schooling and a chance to teach. To free the girls from household responsibility, William Morris married again in 1852 to Ellen R. Thomas in Canton, Ohio. She was a congenial companion for the rest of his life.

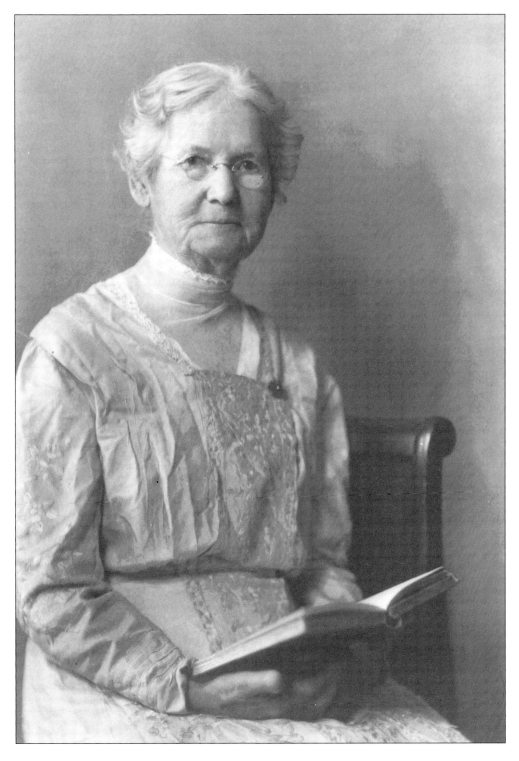

Adaline Morris Larimore (1839-1934), maternal grandmother of Lois Pendleton.

Kate, Jane, and Adaline could now follow their brother Milton as pupils of Alfred Holbrook. He was then teaching at Marlborough, where Kate became a student. In 1855 Holbrook established the Southwestern State Normal School at Lebanon, Ohio, near Cincinnati. There Kate, Jane, and Adaline studied and enjoyed the most inspiring years of their lives. This pioneer in teacher-training furnished board, room, and instruction at a price that country teachers could afford, when their pay was rarely more than a dollar a day. Holbrook and his wife, Melissa, managed to furnish board and room at $2.25 a week. Classes were held from seven in the morning to eight or nine in the evening. Enthusiasm for learning was intense.

Holbrook was also concerned with the health of his pupils; he bought gymnasium equipment and croquet sets. Then he organized baseball teams (the game was new in the 1850's). A firm believer in co-education, he encouraged the women to participate. "The young ladies, in sun bonnets and gloves, were permitted to form separate nines or to join the nines of the young men." Eventually Holbrook gave up these sports teams and decided that long walks to and from school, as well as the dashes between classes, furnished exercise enough. There were also botanical and bird-study excursions. Holbrook said, "The wholesome mingling of the sexes was an advantage to health."

Kate became a capable teacher and became the principal of the high school at Mansfield, Ohio, where she married John Henry Reed, superintendent.

During these years William Morris kept busy with his farm and his duties as justice of the peace; he was now Squire Morris. He had with him and Ellen the two youngest girls, Sarah and Dosia. After 1856 he also raised four children of Lewis's widow; she died of tuberculosis, leaving Josephine, Solon, Mary, and Elizabeth. William undertook the care of all of them after raising eleven of his own. He died March 14, 1861, at age 68 and was buried in the cemetery at New Franklin, Ohio.

Adaline married a railroad man named Edwin Moore in 1860 in Bryan, Ohio, where she had lived and taught school, not far from Frank in northwestern Ohio. They had one child, Morris Ellsworth Moore (1861 to 1922). After her husband's death in a railroad accident a few years after their marriage, Adaline married Dr. Andrew Jackson Larimore, a physician in general practice in Bryan, Ohio, who was born January 21, 1815 in Boone County, Indiana. He was a widower with three children: Ford, Mary and Belle.

Dr. Larimore and Adaline had three more children of their marriage: John A. Larimore (d. 1922) who became a leading lawyer in Minneapolis and President of the Minnesota Bar Association; Jessie (May 10, 1870 to January 1948) a school teacher in Minneapolis who married John Louis Pendleton on June 25, 1889; and Jennie (d. 1919) who married Charles Lawton.

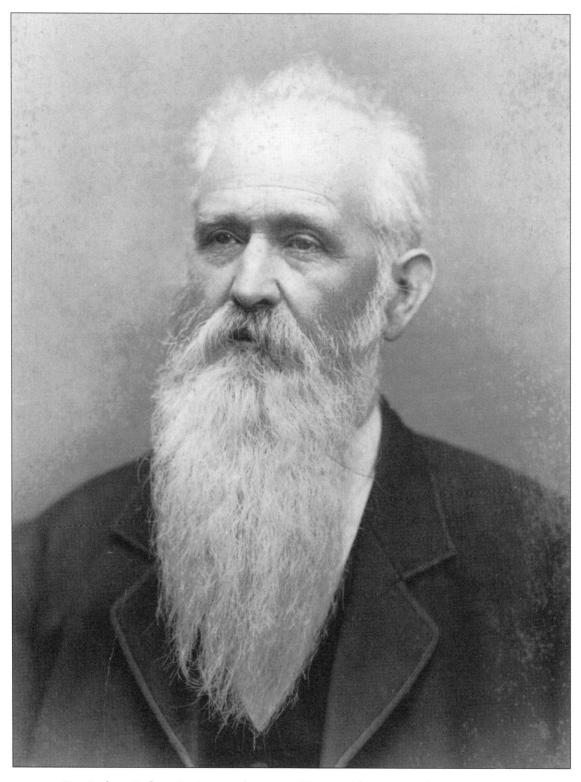

Dr. Andrew Jackson Larimore, physician of Bryan, Ohio, pictured in 1875.
Maternal grandfather of Lois Pendleton.

Adaline was kept busy caring for a large and complicated family of children and step-children. "His children, her children, and our children" were all united into one family as brothers and sisters—there never were any distinctions between them. She had a fine, independent mind. A true philosopher, she observed life and accepted it. This helped her survive the loss of a second husband. Dr. Larimore died suddenly of a stroke while visiting his son, Ford, in Oklahoma. After moving northwest to Minneapolis, she opened a boarding house to support herself and her children.

Adaline made her home with her daughter Jessie and John Louis Pendleton after they moved to California, becoming part of their family in Saratoga, Berkeley, and Los Angeles. She moved with her daughter Jessie and her namesake granddaughter, Adaline, to Claremont after the death of Jessie's husband. She continued to live with them until her death in 1934 at the age of 95. (Her spinning wheel and little rocking chair were saved by the family for her granddaughter, Dr. Adaline Pendleton Satterthwaite.)

A sympathetic listener, a helping hand, and comforter, she read many stories to the Pendleton children and played games with them, like tic-tac-toe and anagrams. She was a wise, comforting, and very understanding person.

JESSIE LARIMORE PENDLETON

Jessie was born in Bryan, Ohio, on May 10, 1870, to Adaline Ann Morris Moore Larimore and Dr. Andrew Jackson Larimore, a beloved physician in Bryan. It was a second marriage for both Adaline and Dr. Larimore, widow and widower.

Jessie was the middle child of the three from the marriage of Adaline and Dr. Larimore. She became a teacher at age eighteen, after graduating from high school and after one year of teacher training. Jessie taught school in Minneapolis and her brother, John, studied law at the University of Minnesota.

One of the young single men who rented a room at her mother's boarding house was John Louis Pendleton. Jessie and J. Louis Pendleton both participated in the Christian Endeavor group at the Plymouth Congregational Church in Minneapolis and soon fell in love. They were married in this church June 25, 1889, when Jessie was nineteen years old. Their first two children were born in Minneapolis.

They moved west because of his health to Saratoga, California, in 1895, with their two small children: Robert Larimore Pendleton (b. June 25, 1890) and Lois Pendleton (b. April 14, 1894). During the Saratoga years two more children were born to Jessie and Louis: Morris Blanchard (b. February 4, 1901) and David Andrew (b. August 21, 1909; d. 1914). Their last child, Adaline (b. February 7, 1917) was born after the family moved to Berkeley.

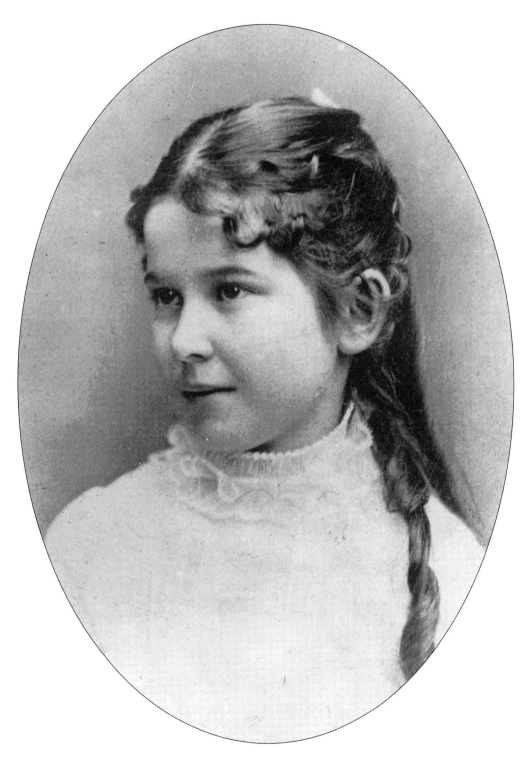

Jessie Larimore age 10 in 1880.

Jessie's talents included a good mastery of Latin. She could figure out the meaning of almost any word from its Latin derivation. Gifted in music, perhaps from her Welsh ancestry through the the Morris family, she had a lovely rich alto voice. She sang in church choirs and oratorio choruses, played the piano, and conducted the church choir for a time in Saratoga. Jessie was outgoing, social, and gregarious. An avid letter writer, she kept in touch regularly with her children: Robert in India, the Philippines, and Thailand; with Lois in China (1920 to 1938); and later with Adaline in Puerto Rico and also in China. Jessie also corresponded with many relatives all across America.

FAMILY FOUNDATIONS III

Saratoga History

(Extensive quotations from *Saratoga's First Hundred Years* by Florence R. Cunningham, copyright 1967, Saratoga Historical Foundation.)

Saratoga, situated along the western border of Santa Clara Valley south of San Francisco was a frontier town. Mineral springs located a mile up the canyon above Saratoga were discovered in the early 1850's. When chemical ingredients of the mineral water were found to be almost identical with those of Congress Springs, one of the larger fountains at a spa at Saratoga, New York, the name Saratoga was chosen for the new town by popular vote on October 6, 1864. Pacific Congress Springs spa opened in 1866, frequented by wealthy visitors and investors from San Francisco.

Saratoga is located in the Thermal Belt. "The warm air of the valley rising at night along the mountain sides, meets the currents flowing in over the mountains, and this is formed into an eddy which hugs the land and wards off the colder temperatures." The area is practically exempt from frost. The salubrious climate made the gardens showcases of floral beauty. Fruit orchards flourished.

In the 1880's many newcomers were beginning to settle in Saratoga. "While they represented a wide range of backgrounds, they had one bond in common; they were coming to Saratoga to grow fruit despite the opinion of 'wise-acres' who said it could not be done."

AGRICULTURE IN SARATOGA

"Large tracts of uncultivated land and partially cleared land were available. The task of tilling partially cleared land was arduous, back-breaking drudgery. Huge oak and sycamore stumps with giant suckers, other large trees and dense thickets of brush and poison oak had to be removed. Poor equipment made it a difficult chore. First, a heavy gang plow (pulled by horses) ripped the chaparral loose and as much of it as possible was gathered up with horse-drawn rakes. Women and children followed behind the rakes gathering the broken, scattered roots and limbs. Many an acreage was a family business with each member doing his share of the work. This was not all the women and children did. Other brush and many rocks had to be gathered. Orchard loam minus rocks was a lot more comfortable on the children's knees as they crawled over the ground when picking prunes."

After the ground was cleared, the men dug holes and planted the fruit trees. Later, the ground around the trees had to be hoed, and as the trees grew larger and were pruned, there were clippings to pick up. "Any tasks that could be done by the women and children released the men folks for the heavier, harder orchard duties."

Older settlers of Saratoga were converting their hay and grain fields to fruit orchards. With the growing demand for fruit trees the price of nursery stock soared. "Some of the early fruit growers solved this problem by raising seedlings that they later grafted and budded."

"Quite a number of the newcomers were people of limited means who had put their all into their land, and some even had to go in debt. It would be several years before there were any crops and even small financial returns. Meanwhile, they and their families must eat and, if in debt, it behooved them to get their land paid for as soon as possible. Therefore work of any sort was eagerly sought, and even though living costs were lower than now, the wages were most meager, a good wage being $1.50 per day, or 15 cents an hour. At Dr. George Handy's big ranch (Glen Una) one of the earliest prune crops was sold on the trees to a prominent San Jose firm. In harvesting they paid only $1.25 for an eleven hour day, 50 cents additional being paid if the men could furnish a horse. This huge orchard was, for a number of years, a source of needed employment for several of these struggling fruit growers."

"While growing fruit was still in an experimental stage, the early-day growers experienced great anxiety waiting for the first fruit to ripen. No one knew what fruits would do best in the various soils, what would have the greatest market appeal or bring the best prices. Because of this uncertainty, a large variety of fruits were planted." The most successful fruit was the lowly French prune, introduced by Louis Pellier (d.1872), the triumph of his prized "la petit prune d'Agen".

With the first harvests came the problem of marketing. Evaporators and driers were built to preserve the fruit. "Time and experience proved that both pitted fruit and lye-dipped prunes could be sun dried with safety and little expense. Then most of the growers, even those with small acreages, began to dry their fruit before selling it, which brought them better prices."

"In 1866, the United States imported 11,048,477 pounds of dried prunes from Europe. Soon the situation reversed itself, and by 1890 the fruit boom was well underway." By 1892 more than half the prunes trees in America were growing in Santa Clara County.

"Prune season extended usually from August through September. After the prunes were picked from the ground, mainly by the younger generation, they were brought to the dipper and drier. Few indeed were the children of that day who did not experience the back-breaking, but valuable (and unappreciated) discipline of picking prunes. When nature decided that the prune was ready to pick, it simply dropped from the tree. Then the children crawled around on the ground, picking the fallen fruit which they placed in buckets, and later emptied into 40-pound boxes. Denim overalls with pads about four inches thick stitched to the knees were worn by the pickers; otherwise the knees would be badly bruised from the rough clods or small stones. But, oh how big those dollars looked after laboriously earning them by picking prunes at five cents a box!"

"Light wagons drawn by teams of horses hauled the filled and stacked boxes from the orchard to the processing area. Here the prunes were dipped in boiling lye solution to crack the skin, and then they were run through a shaker onto the trays for drying in the sun. Prunes underwent a reducing course under the hot sun rays, and finally emerged a figure of wrinkles. Later they were scraped from the trays, graded and marketed." The fruit trays were each four by eight feet and made of white wood.

"If rain threatened during the prune drying season the growers aided by the families and neighbors, rushed to the drying yards and stacked trays as high as two men could lift them. Two empty trays were set at an angle on top of the stack making a slanting roof. Then if rain did come, it would run off the roof instead of seeping down into the half-dry prunes."

"After prunes and grapes, the next fruit of importance to Saratoga growers was the apricot. While there are several varieties of apricots, the Blenheim was best adapted to Saratoga climate, as well as best for canning and drying."

"In the earlier decades of the fruit industry, practically all the community including the women and children looked forward to the fruit harvest as an economic advantage. It was the main source of earning pin money for the children, which was usually spent for clothes, toys and amusements." Picking prunes and cutting apricots "provided a sociable summer in the orchard or the cutting shed".

"Apricot cutters in the late nineties and the turn of the century were paid about 8 cents per box. The majority of farmers dried their own apricots. A work shed was provided for the workers with tables or carpenter horses holding the trays. These were placed at a convenient height for a woman's standing or reaching ability. Apricots were first cut in half, pitted and spread on these trays cut side up, were later sulphured and placed in the drying yard to sun-dry before they hit the market. Later the fruit was scraped from the trays, graded, boxed and stored in the fruit house and eventually delivered to the processor. Cut fruit was never left overnight without sulphuring; otherwise it lost its color and darkened."

"Cutting apricots provided a hilarious summer of fun for many youngsters. Usually a grower's wife worked in the cutting shed, acting as 'floor lady,' keeping an eye on the workers. Larger sheds required a special kind of genius to keep things operating effectively. 'Floor ladies' were placed in strategic positions to ward off the impending mischief. Each cutter had a numbered card, which was punched for each box of cut apricots. Constant vigilance was necessary. Mothers had to keep children from sneaking off for a ride on the supply truck or playing practical jokes on one another. Occasionally someone would throw an apricot pit, and the 'target' would suspect a certain individual. Then he would retaliate with a large mushy apricot and the 'war was on.' Other youngsters preferred more orderly amusement. They would tell stories in a round fashion with one starting a story and others in turn adding their individual bit to the plot. -- Pretty girls flirted with the supply boys hoping to get larger fruit. The larger the fruit, the quicker one could finish cutting a box. The constant chant of 'Tray, please' and 'Box, please' was heard in every voice range. One met quite a cross section of personalities in the cutting shed."

"Not only did Saratoga pioneer fruit growing, but it also had the world's largest prune orchard, Glen Una, located about halfway between Saratoga and Los Gatos. Glen Una, a model self-sufficient farm, with its private water works, electric power plant, paint shed, blacksmith shop, brought fame and distinction to Saratoga, not only for its size, but also for its perfection in every aspect from its carefully pruned and cultivated trees to the artistic lettering of its resplendent fruitwagons. The residence and packing houses were connected with Los Gatos, and all the principal towns in the State, by a long-distance telephone. The fifteen acre plat used as a drying ground was equipped with electric lights. All work involving the handling and packing of the dried fruit was done at night to avoid particles of dust (from the dirt roads) settling on the fruit which sometimes happens during the days." Two rows of incandescent lamps lighted the entire length of the packing house. The drying yard was a hundred feet below the packing house. At the peak of the harvest season there were sometimes as many as 18,000 white wooden fruit trays, each four by eight feet, drying in the sun. The miles of graveled, sprinkled roads were constantly repaired by Glen Una's own crews and its own sprinkling wagons. Water was piped from the springs to every building on the ranch under a pressure of 150 pounds to the square inch. A hose cart, filled from water towers on the ranch, provided fire protection."

"The lowly prune now emerged as a fruit with a wealth of nutritional charm." Santa Clara County became "French prune mad," and in 1889 captured the fruit market everywhere: London, Paris, New York. "In 1890 Santa Clara County had 6175 acres of prunes, but by 1900 the County had 35,701 acres, and the State's acreage was around 90,000. Plantings continued steadily, and in 1925 the County had 62,296 acres of bearing prunes and 4245 acres of non-bearing."

"What made these Saratoga orchards noteworthy was the fact that the owners had planted that still far from popular fruit (in the 1870's), the French prune." It was now twenty years since Pierre and John Pellier had brought to their brother, Louis, those "two treasure trunks" full of cuttings and scions, for which they had scouted France at his request. Nothing in these two trunks was more prized by Louis than the few scions of "la petit prune d'Agen." He had recognized the similarity of the soil and climate of Santa Clara Valley to the soil and climate of the French homeland of this fruit, so highly rated in Europe. Stuck into potatoes and carefully packed in sawdust to retain the proper moisture during the long sea voyage, the scions had arrived in perfect condition. Their skillfully effected grafts soon proved "naturals." Louis Pellier, born in France in 1817, came to Santa Clara Valley in 1849-50. He was so enchanted with the beauty and climate that he bought a small acreage in San Jose, which soon became a community showplace attracting people from great distances to see his garden and orchard. Pellier introduced the first prune graftings to Santa Clara County. Unfortunately he didn't live to see the fabulous growth of the prune industry.

"About the same time Saratoga was beginning to plant orchards, a number of vineyards were planted in the sloping hills above town. The sunny southern exposure with the chalky clay soil, caused the vines to grow in a remarkable way and the grapes to acquire a flavor never imparted by valley soil. Some divided their land between prunes, apricots and grapes." One of the world's most celebrated vineyards with picturesque sandstone winery, the famed Paul Masson's "vineyard in the sky," is located on Pierce Road on a steep hillside above Saratoga.

SARATOGA CHURCHES

"Many of the families settling here were church-going people with hearts opened to God. When they found no church of their particular denomination, they set about organizing one. Thus the Congregational Church became the first permanent religious organization in the town. With a charter membership of nine women and one man, it began its long years of Christian service on June 2, 1872. Because there was no Congregational Church in San Jose at that time, Rev. E. M. Betts, pastor of the new school First Presbyterian Church in San Jose, held the inspiring inaugural services. And, students from the Pacific Theological Seminary, officiated at occasional services until a resident pastor was appointed in 1875."

"There was a true feeling of Christian fellowship in the community with diversified groups working for everyone's welfare. It seemed only natural for the Congregational pastor to announce the strawberry social at the Christian Church or for the Methodist pastor to recommend attendance at the concert sponsored by the Congregationalists. When there was a fifth Sunday in the month, the three churches with resident pastors, Congregational, Christian and Methodist, held their customary evening services as a joint affair, led by the Women's Temperance Union, using the three church buildings in rotation."

"After the turn of the century, talk of church consolidation began partly on recollection of many instances of interdenominational cooperation in the past." In 1919 "an invitation was issued to each of the Protestant churches to meet and draw out a plan of consolidation. The Episcopalians declined because of doctrinal differences, the Methodists on advice of higher Conference authority. This left the Congregational and Christian Churches to come together as the Saratoga Federated Church. This was achieved after lengthy sessions, fortified by the wise counsel of respective pastors. The same silver-toned bell (of the Congregational Church) that brought much enjoyment to the community of yore summons the congregation of the Federated Church to worship today."

"Throughout the town's history the churches maintained their importance as centers of cultural and social as well as spiritual life."

CLUBS OF SARATOGA

Prominent clubs in Saratoga before the turn of the century included the Saratoga Village Improvement Association (1887), a local Woman's Christian Temperance Union, and a local Chautauqua Circle (1886). The Saratoga Village Improvement Association was the town's first booster organization and the forerunner of many of the Improvement Associations, Boards of Trade, and Chamber of Commerce and any other group who worked together for the community's welfare. It was the prime mover in the road sprinkling experiment to keep down the dust. It was "organized for the purpose of acquiring suitable tracts of land, subdividing it into ten-acre lots to be sold on easy terms. When purchased the owner would start improving his land using one acre for a residence and the remaining nine acres would remain under the control of the company subject to terms of sale until the orchards became fruit bearing and final payments made. The object of the Association was to beautify the roads by planting shade trees, sprinkling roads and streets, grading and maintaining roads, planting hedges, encouraging social intercourse by lectures and similar programs, promote order, tidiness and all other features conducive to the health and property of Saratoga and vicinity."

Officers of the Saratoga Village Improvement Association were:
President: Milton H. Myrick, Ex-Supreme Court Justice (State)
Vice-President: James E. Gordon
Vice-President: Jennie M. Farwell
Recording Secretary: L. A. Sage
Corresponding Secretary: Carrie H. Gordon
Treasurer: Frank M. Farwell

Franklin M. Farwell (1834-1903) was "Saratoga's beloved and outstanding pioneer" who came to the future site of Saratoga in 1856. "For five years he mined for gold in the Sierra and Nevada Counties before returning. Except for a seven year period in the 1870's when in business in San Francisco, he spent the remainder of his life on the Farwell Ranch, Bella Vista (now the Kirkwood estate). Although a busy rancher, he was a dedicated and enthusiastic community leader supporting every project with high ideals for the betterment of Saratoga until his death in 1903. Some of his affiliations include the Congregational Church, Improvement Club, school trustee, Madronia Cemetery Association, road sprinkling development, Blossom Festival and the Saratoga Missionary Settlement." He lived with his sister Miss Jennie Farwell at their homestead on Rancho Bella Vista. Frank and Jennie were both outstanding citizens active in the betterment of the community.

Palo Alto Times

"THE OTHER HALF" by Cornelia Matijasevich
December 7, 1954

DR. LOIS TODD COMBINES TWO CAREERS

Professionally she's Dr. Lois Pendleton Todd, but in private life she's Mrs. Oliver Julian Todd, wife of the world-famed civil engineer who put China's Yellow River back into its right course.

To some—mainly the Chinese—Oliver Todd is known as Todd the River Tamer, because he has done more to harness the Yellow River than any other man in history—to his contemporaries he's affectionately called "Todd Almighty."

To all—especially Stanford students—Mrs. Todd is known only as Doctor Todd.

Since receiving her medical degree at the University of California Medical School in 1920, the former Lois Pendleton has been practicing medicine, only taking time out to bring up a family of four—two girls and two boys—during those years making eight trips across the Pacific between the United States and China.

On completing medical school and internship in 1920 she went to China to practice medicine.

Why did she go to China? As she put it: "I realized the great need for physicians trained in western medicine, and particularly the need for women physicians. I studied medicine because I loved it and wanted to work where I thought I could do the most good."

So, from 1920 to 1927 young Dr. Pendleton had seven years of very concentrated medical and surgical work at Williams-Porter Hospital in Tehchow, Shantung, China.

However, the first six months were spent in Peking at the College of Chinese Studies—learning the language.

Thereafter, full medical responsibilities were assumed and language study continued a couple of hours a day so that at the end of five years she received her five year diploma from the College.

Whether it was asking for an instrument in the operating room, or directiong the care of patients, her work had to be carried out in the Chinese language—for her nurses knew little English.

Then in March 1927—in the midst of her busy life—the summons came from the U.S. Consular representative for all women and children to leave the interior stations. This was due to the Nanking Incident of the Nationalist Revolution.

During these days of waiting for a sailing in Tientsin, Oliver Todd, a young engineer, an alumnus from the University of Michigan, came into her life.

At the time of their meeting Mr. Todd had already served as an assistant engineer with the City of San Francisco and was captain of engineers in World War I—having been cited by General Pershing for meritorious service, and now was directing the use of famine labor in building the first motor roads in Shantung Province.

"He came north," said Dr. Todd, "on so-called urgent business and that evening before I sailed for the Philippines we became engaged."

After two months they were married in the tropical garden at Los Banos College—home of her brother, Robert L. Pendleton, who is now a professor at Johns Hopkins University and considered the leading soils technologist in the world.

In the fall of 1927 they established their home in Peking, which remained their home for the 11 succeeding years.

Their four children were all born in Peking, and it was during those years Dr. Todd limited her practice so that she could devote much time to her family.

Their four children were bilingual from the start; talking to the servants in Chinese and to their parents in English.

There was nothing I could do to induce them to use Chinese, much to their regret later on, she said.

Of the four, the two girls went into medicine—following their mother's footsteps; and the two boys have gone into engineering.

Their older daughter, Dr. Doris Todd Brown, is married to David P. Brown of San Francisco. They have two daughters—the Todds' only two grandchildren.

The Todds' younger daughter, Mrs. Robert M. Christiansen (Elinor Todd) is a senior at Women's Medical College in Philadelphia and will receive her M.D. Degree in June.

James Pendleton Todd, their older son, received his master's degree in mechanical engineering at Stanford and is now a test engineer at the Pratt-Whitney Airplane Factory in East Hartford, Connecticut.

Hewlett, youngest of the four Todd children, is a senior at Cal Poly, where he is studying agricultural engineering. He was married during the summer to the former Susan Swig of Honolulu.

While the children were young, Dr. Todd found time to help her husband in proof reading on the books he wrote.

In the "Chinese Bronze Mirrors" she also aided, with the essential help of a Chinese scholar who could decipher the ancient "grass characters," succeed in translating the inscriptions on the ancient bronze mirrors.

Between 1920 and 1938 Dr. Todd made the eight trips across the Pacific all by boat. She recalls how different the first trips were in comparison with the busy ones when there were four little children to watch—ranging in age from 5 to 10 years.

The Japanese invasion of North China forced Major Todd to give up his engineering work in 1938—the year they settled in Palo Alto.

"I always knew Palo Alto would be a fine place to bring up a family," said Dr. Todd.

The Deep Peninsula was not new territory to this young homemaker. Although she was born in Minneapolis her family moved to Saratoga when she was a very young girl.

She recalls her school-girl days, when she rode horseback 12 miles each day, back and forth from her home in Saratoga to Campbell Union High School, from where she was graduated.

In the fall after their return to the Peninsula Dr. Todd started part time work with Dr. Helen Pryor on the Women's Health Service at Stanford and since 1940 she has been full time physician on the Health Service.

Dr. Todd was the only physician on the two services who was employed in the new set-up. She is also the only full-time woman physician on the present staff.

Although she has devoted much time to her medical work, her children were being trained at home, so that they could become familiar with the every-day routine, domestic responsibilities.

Each was responsible for certain chores so that they had not only their clothing allowance, but also their small earning to budget. "This experience was helpful in the college years which followed," she said.

What does Dr. Todd think about mixing marriage and careers?
"It's a fine thing to be able to mix both and if two people are mature enough to know their own minds and have mutual respect it makes for a fuller life, pro-viding of course one has the desire and requisite course, health, and strength," she said.

"Instability of the home," she said, "is one of the the biggest factors of broken marriages, and broken marriages are apt to result in more of the same," she continued.

While Mr. Todd was busy "taming the Yellow River" there wasn't much she could do besides caring for the family single-handed during his absence.

This past spring, after the four children were of age and nearly all had achieved their goals, Mr. and Mrs. Todd took their "second honeymoon" and went to Europe on a two-month trip; her first to the Continent and his first return trip since the days he spent there in World War I.

Glossary

A.B.C.F.M.—American Board of Commissioners for Foreign Missions, Congregational Church (later United Church of Christ).

ALS—amyotrophic lateral sclerosis (Lou Gehrig's disease)

amah—live-in baby sitter, nanny, or nurse maid.

coolie—native unskilled laborer.

honey pot—jar of human excrement.

ho—river.

hutong—alley.

Kung Li Hui—North China Mission of A.B.C.F.M.

li (le)—a Chinese unit of measure equal to about one third of a mile.

mafoo—horse attendent or helper.

magistrate—a public civil officer, official rank in government.

pagoda—a tower-like structure, usually a temple or a memorial.

pai lo—decorative gateway across an entrance, or in old Peking over a major intersection.

Peking cart—small two wheeled wooden cart, without springs or a seat, pulled by a donkey or mule and used for transporting people.

ricksha—small two wheeled cart with a seat and hood and two long handles pulled by a man running.

P.U.M.C.—Peking Union Medical College (built and endowed by the Rockefeller Foundation in the early 1920's), the first school teaching western medicine in China.

shan—sacred mountain.

t'ang huler—glazed crabapples on a scewer.

U.C.C.—United Church of Christ (established by a merger of Congregational and Evangelical and Reformed churches).

U.N.R.R.A.—United Nations Relief and Rehabilitation Agency, established following World War II.

yamen—in China, the official headquarters or residence of a magistrate or public official.

REFERENCES AND RESOURCES

CHAPTER 1. WESTWARD MOVE
>Narrative from Morris B. Pendleton
>Narrative from Lois Pendleton Todd
>Family photograph albums.

CHAPTER 2. SARATOGA CHILDHOOD
>*Saratoga's First Hundred Years* by Florence R. Cunningham, Saratoga Historical Foundation, 1967, Harlan-Young Press, San Jose, CA 95106
>Narration and letters by Jessie L. Pendleton
>Narration and memories of Lois Pendleton Todd
>Narration and memories of Morris B. Pendleton
>Family photograph albums

CHAPTER 3. BERKELEY STUDENT YEARS
>Narration and memories of Lois Pendleton Todd
>Narration and memories of Morris B. Pendleton
>Family photograph albums

CHAPTER 4. SURGEON IN TEHCHOW
>Letters of Dr. Lois Pendleton
>Letters of Jessie L. Pendleton
>Narration and memories of Dr. Adaline Pendleton Satterthwaite
>Weekly letters of Alice Reed to her family
>Memories of Dr. Arthur Tucker

CHAPTER 5. WEDDING AND KWEICHOW
>Narration of Dr. Adaline Pendleton Satterthwaite
>Letters of Dr. Lois Pendleton
>Diary of Oliver Julian Todd

CHAPTER 6. PEKING FAMILY YEARS
>Diary of Oliver Julian Todd
>Letters of Dr. Lois Pendleton Todd
>Family letters and photograph albums
>Memories of Elinor Todd Christiansen

CHAPTER 7. PALO ALTO: BALANCING CAREER AND FAMILY
    Diary of Oliver Julian Todd
    Letters of Lois Pendleton Todd
    Memories of the Todd children
    Newspaper articles from "The Palo Alto Times"
    Stanford University Faculty Senate Memorial Resolution: LOIS
        PENDLETON TODD

CHAPTER 8. SUNSET YEARS
    Diary of Oliver Julian Todd
    Letters of Lois Pendleton Todd
    Memories of the Todd children

I. NEW ENGLAND ROOTS—The Pendletons
    Brian Pendleton and His Descendents1599-1910
        Compiled by Everett Hall Pendleton
        Privately printed, 1911.
    Early New England Pendletons
        Compiled by Everett Hall Pendleton
        Privately printed, 1956.
    Later New England Pendletons
        A record of the Pendleton family from the 7th to the 12th
        generation
        Compiled by Everett Hall Pendleton
        Privately printed, 1966.
    Sea Captains of Searsport
        author unknown
    Penobscot Marine Museum in Searsport, Maine
        Box 403 D (207) 548-2529

II. PENNSYLVANIA ROOTS—The Morrises
    William Morris and His Family
        Recollections, family stories, and genealogy research compiled
        by Mary Embleton in the 1940's at the suggestion of her cousin
        Lois Pendleton Todd. Mary Embleton was a grand-daughter of
        William Morris.

INDEX

Order Form

Order extra copies of

Doctor Lois

TODAY!

- *A gift for a friend*
  - *A motivational book for teenagers*
    - *An intriguing book for readers interested in China*
      - *A guide for women combining career and family*

Mail Orders To:
Doctor Lois Book Offer
c/o Christiansen
4081 South Holly Street
Denver, CO 80111

Please mail Doctor Lois to the address below:

Name_____

Address_____

City_____State_____Zip_____

_____copies of *Doctor Lois* in the hardcover edition @ 24.95 $_____

_____copies of *Doctor Lois* in the paperback edition @ 16.95 $_____

Tax (Colorado residents only @ 3% .48 paperbk./.75 hardbk. each) $_____

Shipping and handling @ $2 per book $_____

TOTAL ENCLOSED $_____